Biological Therapeutics

Biological Therapeutics

Ben Greenstein PhD, MRPharms
Honorary Visiting Senior Research Fellow, Royal Free Hospital, London, UK.

Daniel A Brook MA, MRCP, MRCGP, DCH
General Practitioner, London, UK

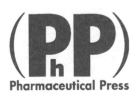

London • Chicago **Pharmaceutical Press**

Published by Pharmaceutical Press

1 Lambeth High Street, London SE1 7JN, UK

1559 St. Paul Avenue, Gurnee, IL 60031, USA

© Royal Pharmaceutical Society of Great Britain 2011

(**P.P**) is a trade mark of Pharmaceutical Press

Pharmaceutical Press is the publishing division of the
Royal Pharmaceutical Society of Great Britain

First published 2011

Typeset by Thomson Digital, Noida, India
Printed in Great Britain by TJ International, Padstow, Cornwall

ISBN 978 0 85369 843 2

A catalogue record for this book is available from the British Library.

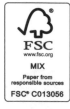

FSC
www.fsc.org
MIX
Paper from
responsible sources
FSC® C013056

Dedication

To our patient families

Contents

Preface

This book has been written as an introduction to what is arguably the most exciting and fastest-growing branch of medicine at the present time: the use of treatments designed to block key exogenous and endogenous mediators of disease. Notable examples include the vaccines and inhibitors of endogenous mediators of inflammation and carcinogenesis. This principle is far from novel because vaccines against disease have been used for many years. What is relatively new is the availability of the so-called biological preparations (the trans-Atlantic nomenclature is biologic), which target key mediators of inflammation and carcinogenesis. Also remarkable is the efficacy and extended half-lives of these drugs, e.g. rituximab, which needs to be given but once a year for rheumatoid arthritis. They are not cures, but they do slow the rate of progression of diseases such as rheumatoid arthritis and extend the useful life of hands, feet and several other joints.

Each chapter begins, where relevant, with a brief historical introduction, followed by an overview of the drugs, their mechanisms of action, uses and examples of adverse reactions already noted. Clinical scenarios appear in some chapters and should help to bring alive the raison d'être of the book.

Chapter 1 deals with the genetic code and introduces some of the key methods used in gene manipulation. Chapter 2 is an account of the vaccines, which, arguably, were the first modern biological drugs. Chapter 3 is a summary of the hormone and hormone-related drugs. Chapter 4 covers basic principles and mechanisms of inflammation, and Chapter 5 introduces the reader to the sphere of autoimmunity, including the phenomenon of immunological tolerance and transplant rejection. Chapter 6 introduces the use of biological drugs, using two important inflammatory diseases caused by autoimmunity, notably rheumatoid arthritis and systemic lupus erythematosus. These are addressed in the context of autoimmunity together with important examples of the biological drugs used.

Chapter 7 deals with the biological antineoplastic drugs, particularly with reference to the epidermal growth factor receptor, which is currently the most important target for these compounds. Finally, Chapter 8 considers stem cell technology and its current and potential use. All the chapters except the final one have a series of multiple choice questions (MCQs) with an answer section after the final chapter.

Best practice and knowledge are constantly changing as new experience and research broaden our knowledge and changes in practice, treatment and drug therapy may be appropriate. Readers should consult the most recent and up-to-date information regarding dose, formulation, precautions and contra-indications provided by regulatory authorities and by manufacturers and suppliers of products they intend to use or prescribe. It is the responsibility of the prescribers, relying on their experience and knowledge of the patient, to make diagnoses, to determine dosages and the best individual treatment for each patient and to take appropriate safety precautions. To the fullest extent of the law, neither the Publisher nor the Authors, assume any liability for any injury and/or damage to persons or property arising out of or related to the use of any material contained in this book.

The book has been designed and written for a very disparate audience. This is a relatively new and fast-growing branch of medicine that will need to be integrated into several undergraduate and postgraduate syllabi and also into the armoury of those who prescribe and dispense these preparations.

BDG
DAB
October 2010

About the authors

Ben Greenstein originally qualified as a pharmacist in South Africa, where he worked mainly in rural areas before immigrating to the UK to work for 3 years as a community pharmacist. He obtained a PhD in Pharmacology at the University of London in 1975 and lectured in Pharmacology at the University of London for 18 years, after which he decided to devote himself to the writing of textbooks in his areas of expertise. He is currently an Honorary Visiting Senior Research Fellow in the Pain Management Service at the Royal Free Hospital, Hampstead, London.

Daniel Brook qualified in 2001, after undergraduate studies at St Catharine's College, Cambridge and Imperial College School of Medicine, London. He trained as a hospital physician in London, gaining the membership to The Royal College of Physicians, before transferring into general practice. He works as a general practitioner with local involvement in undergraduate training in north London.

1

Introduction to genetic manipulation

Objectives:

- Know what is meant by the genetic code and be able to give examples of the code.
- Be aware of the basics of the nomenclature used to describe the code, e.g. codon, deoxynucleotide, nucleotide, gene, purine, pyrimidine, double helix, hydrogen bonding.
- Be able to list the basic sequence from transcription to protein.
- Know what is meant by recombinant DNA technology.
- Explain, in brief, the key processes involved in gene manipulation.
- List some practical applications of recombinant DNA technology.
- Understand the nature of the plasmid and its use as a vector.
- Give examples of viral vector systems.
- Explain what is meant by a restriction endonuclease and, briefly, how it is used.
- Give at least one example of a knockout mouse.

Medicines have been made from plants, animal tissues and minerals, and possibly date back to and conceivably predate the earliest human cultures. Some animals, e.g. cats, are known to seek out certain plants when not well. Hints of herbal or medicinal practice are thought to date back to about 25 000 BC. Early hieroglyphics suggest that Egyptians and Babylonians practised surgery and medicine at least 2500 years ago. Evidence for herbal medicine in Pakistan has been dated back to about 3000 BC and Ayuverdic medicine in India is at least 2000 years old. The Chinese have been practising herbal medicine and acupuncture for at least 5000 years and are known to have practised inoculation against smallpox before 200 BC. Hippocrates (about 460–370 BC), however, is generally accepted in the west as the father of modern medicine, although arguably the most influential early practitioners were the Arab doctors and pharmacists of the first millennium AD, who laid the foundations for the sciences of, for example pharmacology, modern surgery and the quantification of drug effects. Europe, alas, sank into a mediaeval 'Dark Age' of medicine, where for centuries the leech and bloodletting reigned supreme until the Enlightenment of the eighteenth century.

The science of the alteration and manipulation of natural resources to create new chemical compounds is relatively recent in human medical history, and is due mainly to advances in chemical synthesis and medical knowledge. Notable examples include the development of the smallpox and rabies vaccines, and the chemical synthesis of aspirin and its subsequent marketing by the German company Bayer towards the end of the nineteenth century. The discovery and identification of insulin by Banting and Best and their colleagues in the 1920s in Canada marked the birth of endocrinology as a science in its own right, and the consequent saving of thousands, if not millions, of patients with diabetes.

Another very significant advance of the twentieth century was the discovery of the effects of the mould *Penicillium* species on bacteria by Alexander Fleming in 1928, and the subsequent development of penicillin by Florey and Chain in the 1940s. During that decade the introduction of the BCG (Bacille Calmette–Guérin) vaccine and streptomycin offered the first effective treatment for tuberculosis and, in 1944, the first successful heart operation was performed on a baby born with a congenital heart problem, thus ending the previously fatal 'blue baby' birth. The 1950s saw a rapid growth in the development of newer antibiotics and for the first time effective pharmacological tools were available to treat psychiatric patients.

Perhaps the discovery most blessed by patients and healthcare professionals alike was that of the general anaesthetic. Surgery is arguably as old as humanity and so, presumably, is the search for a means of blocking pain during the procedure. The oldest recorded use of morphine for anaesthesia was found in the Egyptian *Ebers Papyrus* around 1552 BC, and from then to the nineteenth century morphine was the mainstay until the discovery of the anaesthetic gases. Analgesia, too, has its roots in the development of biological materials such as morphine and willow bark and the identification of salicylic acid, which eventually led to the synthesis of aspirin. This was followed by a rapid growth of the biological sciences and, of particular relevance to this book, those concerned with amino acids, proteins, RNA, DNA, the elucidation of the genetic code and recombinant DNA technology. Of equal importance was the discovery of the bacterial plasmid, which has become an indispensable tool in the development of many of the new biological therapeutic agents, and also of the structure and function of bacteria and viruses.

Nucleotides and the genetic code

The genetic code (Table 1.1) is a set of biological rules that dictate the translation of genetic information contained within the DNA into specific amino acids and, ultimately, into specific proteins. There are two genetic codes, these being the code for amino acids dictated by the nuclear deoxyribonucleic acid (DNA) and another that is contained within the mitochondria. The code dealt with here is the nuclear one.

The fundamental rule is that each codon consists of three deoxynucleotides, commonly called triplets. There are two classes of deoxyribonucleotides: those containing the purines adenine (A) and guanine (G), and those containing the pyrimidines cytosine (C) and thymine (T). The DNA (this information is limited to eukaryotic DNA) is organised in the form of a double helix formed by the pairing, through hydrogen bonding, of complementary nucleotides represented by A–T and C–G. The DNA is transcribed by the enzyme RNA polymerase to form the corresponding ribonucleic acid (RNA), which is translated by the ribosomes into protein (Figure 1.1).

Table 1.1 The genetic code, showing base code for the amino acids

Second base of codon

First base of the codon	U	C	A	G	Third base of colon
U	UUU UUC Phe / UUA UUG Leu	UCU UCC UCA UCG Ser	UAU UAC Tyr / UAA UAG STOP	UGU UGC Cys / UGA STOP / UGG Trp	U C A G
C	CUU CUC CUA CUG Leu	CCU CCC CCA CCG Pro	CAU CAC His / CAA CAG Gln	CGU CGC CGA CGG Arg	U C A G
A	AUU AUC AUA Ile / AUG Met	ACU ACC ACA ACG Thr	AAU AAC Asn / AAA AAG Lys	AGU AGC Ser / AGA AGG Arg	U C A G
G	GUU GUC GUA GUG Val	GCU GCC GCA GCG Ala	GAU GAC Asp / GAA GAG Glu	GGU GGC GGA GGG Gly	U C A G

Key:
A: adenine
Ala: alanine
Arg: arginine
Asn: asparagine
Asp: aspartate
C: cytosine
Cys: cystine

G: guanosine
Gln: glutamine
Glu: glutamate
Gly: glycine
His: histidine
Ile: isoleucine
Leu: leucine
Lys: lysine
Met: methionine

Phe: phenylalanine
Pro: proline
Ser: serine
STOP: cedon for signal to end translation
Thr: threonine
Trp: tryptophan
U: uracil
Val: valine

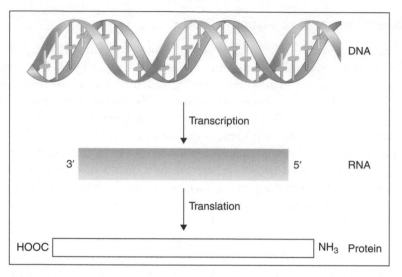

Figure 1.1 Transcription of DNA by the enzyme RNA polymerase to form the corresponding ribonucleic acid (RNA).

It should be noted that the thymine of DNA results in uracil in messenger (m) RNA. The possible number of combinations of triplets is 4^3 or 64.

Recombinant DNA technology

Recombinant DNA technology, also known as genetic engineering or genetic modification, may be defined as the modification of an organism's genes. This science developed from the original discovery of the structure of DNA, the elucidation of the genetic code, and the identification of the genes responsible for the structure and function of the systems necessary for the normal and successful function of a living organism. It has also revolutionised the science of medicine. The traditional chemotherapeutic approach, which relied on the serendipitous identification or synthesis of medicinal compounds, is rapidly being displaced by the production of medicines derived from an understanding of endogenous mediators of, for example, inflammation and carcinogenesis.

Biochemical advances that made possible this relatively new science include the biochemical analysis of proteins and DNA, identification of key mediators of, for example, inflammation, notably tumour necrosis factor-α (TNF-α), and of carcinogenesis, notably the cluster of differentiation (CD) antigens expressed on the cells of the immune system. Key technical advances include the development of methods for the identification and isolation of specific genes coding for gene products of interest, polynucleotide replication *in vitro*, e.g. the polymerase chain reaction (PCR), the science of proteomics which has made available the rapid identification of minute quantities of proteins in, for example, a tiny gel slice, and the invention of plasmid and viral vectors for the *in vitro* mass production of specific gene products.

Methods have also been developed in order to isolate precisely and splice out of the genome the segment of DNA that contains the genetic information to generate specific proteins. These can be inserted into biological factories, e.g. bacterial cells, which will produce large quantities of the desired gene product.

The key processes involved in gene manipulation may be summarised as:

- isolation of the gene under study
- combination of the gene with an appropriate transfer vector, e.g. a plasmid or virus
- introduction of the vector into the system to be modified
- ability to identify the artificially modified organisms and to separate them from organisms not modified
- isolation of the gene of interest.

Practical applications of recombinant DNA technology include the following:

- Genetic modification of crops to confer resistance to disease, improve crop yield and, in some cases, to alter appearance in order to improve visual appeal.
- Identification of desirable or unwanted genes in an attempt to prevent inheritance of, for example, certain heritable diseases. It is not inconceivable that future generations of fetuses will be scanned for the presence of a wide range of these diseases and, through (currently controversial) decisions, these diseases will be eliminated from the species.
- Mass biosynthesis of medicinal products, e.g. hormones such as insulin (the first to be approved by the US Food and Drug Administration [FDA] using this technology) and the *in vitro* synthesis of human growth hormone, previously available only through posthumous human donors.
- The (controversial) creation of genetically modified fruit and vegetables, which, for example, may rot more slowly than their unmodified relations.
- The research into the aetiology of inherited diseases, in the hope that these may ultimately be eliminated through the screening of fetuses within families known to carry the disease.
- Gene knock-out experimentation (see below), an invaluable tool, using genetically modified mice, for elucidating the function of genes with an unknown function.

The tools used for recombinant DNA technology

Assembling and combining DNA from different sources creates recombinant DNA. A desired sequence is usually spliced into another sequence, e.g. that of a plasmid or bacterium, usually for the purpose of amplification of the ultimate product, e.g. insulin by bacteria. The process of amplification and magnification of the yield is called cloning. The term 'clone' refers to an identical copy of the parent.

Plasmid vectors

The plasmid is a fundamental tool for cloning purposes. Plasmids occur naturally in many bacteria as (roughly) circular, self-replicating, extra-chromosomal DNA. They are tools that enable the bacterium to survive and reproduce itself under (sometimes rapidly) changing conditions of the external environment. They confer resistance to threats including anti-biotics and bacteriophages. An example of a plasmid, PBR322, is shown in Figure 1.2.

Plasmids are not considered part of the chromosomal DNA that codes for the proteins. They are important in a therapeutic sense, in that they carry genes that confer resistance to antibiotics. They are important in recombinant DNA technology because the DNA of interest can be spliced into the plasmid by cutting the plasmid DNA at chosen sites using specific restriction nucleases, and inserting the DNA that codes for the wanted protein (e.g. insulin – see below), and then annealing the plasmid to restore its circular structure. The plasmid is inserted into a bacterium, e.g. *Escherichia coli*, which when incubated should, if all is well, produce the desired gene product, in this case insulin.

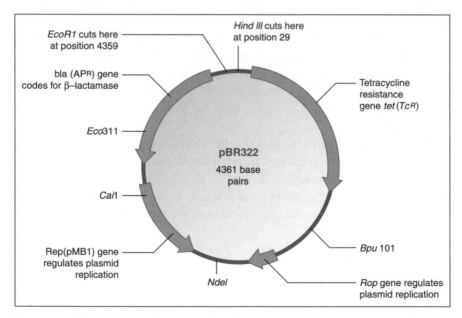

Figure 1.2 Plasmid PBR322 showing sites for selected restriction enzymes (not comprehensive).

The structure of the plasmid must be known absolutely in order to manipulate it. Thus, the nucleotide sequence of PBR322 is fully established.

The Human Genome Project

This was a project aimed at the sequencing of the whole human genome, which was achieved and the results published in 2004. The data have greatly facilitated the identification and study of very many previously unknown genes involved in the differentiation, development and maintenance of the organism. This information also adds a new clinical dimension to the understanding and treatment of disease, especially inherited disease. Furthermore, it is highly likely that it will revolutionise the treatment of disease and (controversially) it will provide prospective parents with a more complete prenatal genetic database.

Viral vectors

Plasmids are not the only vectors used. Viral gene delivery systems are proving to be powerful tools. The virus is first rendered unable to replicate, and such a virus is termed 'recombinant deficiency'. These viruses are used to transmute both dividing and post-mitotic cells and make possible very powerful and easily regulated expression of specific genes. This method is potentially able to allow the introduction of new genes into both developing and adult organisms with improved efficiency, long-term potential, greater reliability and a greatly reduced chance of provoking an immune response in the recipient.

Four main types of viral delivery systems have been developed (at the time of writing):

1 adenovirus
2 recombinant adeno-associated virus (rAAV)
3 herpes simplex virus (HSV)
4 retrovirus.

Adenoviruses are not RNA but DNA viruses responsible for, for example, conjunctivitis and upper respiratory infections. There are at least 45 types of adenovirus and many cause disease, particularly in children and infants.

The rAAV viruses, which belong to the *Parvoviridae* family of viruses, are of particular interest here because they appear to be completely non-pathogenic and are therefore the focus of much interest in the development of therapeutic vectors. Studies have shown that they are highly efficient gene transfer tools that can be used in many human cell types. A single application often results in significantly extended and stable expression of genes introduced into the host tissue.

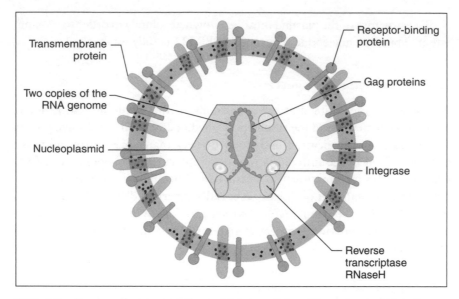

Figure 1.3 Structure of a retrovirus. Gag proteins are proteins of the nucleoplasmid shell around the virus; integrase is the protein of a retrovirus (e.g. HIV) that permits viral genome to be integrated into the host DNA; nucleoplasmid contains the viral pre-genome RNA, the DNA product of which will eventually be spliced into the host cell DNA. (After Howarth JL, Bok-Lee Y, Uney JB. Using viral vectors as gene transfer tools. *Cell Biol Toxicol* 2010;**26**:1–20.)

Herpes simplex virus is well known for infection of mucous membranes, nerves and skin. It is the infective agent for cold sores, fever blisters and some eye infections.

The retroviruses (Figure 1.3) are a family of RNA-based viruses that possess the enzyme reverse transcriptase. Once the virus has penetrated into the host cell, the cell uses the viral reverse transcriptase to produce viral DNA, which is integrated into the host cell DNA. Diseases are transmitted sexually, and a notorious example is the human immunodeficiency virus (HIV).

Restriction endonucleases

Restriction endonucleases are enzymes that digest or cut both single- and double-stranded DNA at specific restriction sites depending on the enzyme used. The enzyme recognises one specific nucleotide sequence and 'cuts' the DNA strand at this point. Many are available, each specific for a certain nucleotide sequence. For example, the enzyme EcoRI cuts double-stranded DNA thus:

G/AATTC
CTTAA/G

The cut plasmid is then incubated together with the DNA strand of interest in the presence of a ligase enzyme, e.g. phage T4 ligase, which forms covalent links between five-carbon phosphate and three-carbon hydroxyl groups, thereby re-forming the closed plasmid circle. Plasmids are not the only vectors used. Liposomes and viruses are commonly used as vectors.

The modified vector must then be inserted into the organism in which it will be amplified through replication of that organism. The bacteria are cultured.

The modified bacterium must then be separated from unmodified organisms. This can be achieved, for example, by conferring resistance to a specific antibacterial agent when the organism takes up the sequence of interest. If the organisms are then exposed to the antibacterial, only the transformed bacteria will survive.

Mass production of insulin: an example

Insulin is a protein normally synthesised by the islet cells of the pancreas, which limits the potentially dangerous build-up of glucose in the blood by promoting glucose uptake into the tissues. In patients with type 1 or juvenile-onset diabetes the islet cells are attacked and destroyed through autoimmune attack by the immune system, leaving patients at risk of potentially fatal hyperglycaemia.

Traditionally, insulin was isolated from animal (mainly porcine) and human pancreata. Porcine insulin carries with it the risk of antibody production by the human immune system, thus lessening or neutralising the beneficial effects of the administered insulin. Furthermore, human insulin could not be reliably obtained. The availability of recombinant DNA technology has guaranteed a reliable and abundant supply of human insulin, which was, to the author's knowledge, the first recombinant medicine produced.

The nature of insulin

Insulin is a comparatively small protein of molecular weight 5808, consisting of two chains connected by two disulphide bridges. Chain A has 30 amino acids and chain B has 21 amino acids. The genetic information for the transcription of insulin mRNA occurs on the short arm of chromosome 11.

Steps in the production of insulin using recombinant DNA technology

In summary:

1   The DNA that codes for insulin is purified and inserted into a plasmid, which is circular DNA isolated from, for example, the bacterium E. coli (see Figure 1.2).

2   The plasmid is enzymatically cut at predetermined sites using restriction enzymes so that the chain is opened.
3   Insulin DNA can be attached to the chain, and the chain is closed again.
4   The resealed, recombinant plasmid is introduced into a bacterium, usually *E. coli*, and the modified *E. coli* will now produce, in culture, human insulin.

It should be mentioned that the strain of *E. coli* used needs to be one that lacks the enzymes that could digest the insulin produced by the bacterial cell.

Knockout mice

Knockout mice are mice with genes that have been experimentally altered so that a specific gene or set of genes has been inactivated or 'switched off' in order to assess the effect on the animal. This technique helps to establish the role of the genes chosen in terms of, for example, immune function and resistance to disease, normal physiological function of organs or behaviour. The mouse is particularly useful in this respect because humans and mice have a remarkable number of genes in common. Very many types of knockout mice are now available.

To engineer a gene knockout mouse, the chosen gene has first to be isolated from the murine gene library and altered experimentally to inactivate it, and in addition is given some form of marker to identify it, e.g. a gene that confers resistance to infection or produces a particular colour in the fur of the genetically altered offspring.

The next step is to extract stem cells from a mouse embryo, and the inactivated gene is inserted into the chromosomes of the stem cells. The altered stem cells are introduced into mouse blastocysts, which are then implanted into the uterine lining of a pregnant mouse. The resultant offspring will have the normal coloured fur or the colouring dictated by the genes of the knockout mouse.

The technology is still relatively young and success rates are highly variable. Genetic manipulation of this nature is still somewhat 'hit and miss', since the results of genetic tinkering are as yet highly unpredictable. Problems include the possibility that the gene may not affect the course or nature of development if inserted at the wrong stage of development, or that the genetic alteration may be compensated for and the gene overruled or ignored by the developing fetus. Nevertheless, the technique does hold interesting, if sometimes controversial, possibilities for, for example, disease prevention, fertility control and longevity.

Controversially and of great interest, at the time of writing, is a highly publicised report from a laboratory of a genetically engineered cell that has spontaneously reproduced itself.

Multiple choice questions

For each question, a maximum of five options is provided and only one is correct.

1 The genetic code dictates the transcription of genetic information directly into:
  a Ribosomal protein
  b Messenger RNA
  c Inheritable traits
  d Ribonucleic acid
  e Intranuclear protein

2 The fundamental rule of the genetic code is that each codon consists of:
  a Three nucleotides
  b Three ribosomes
  c Chromosomal RNA
  d Three deoxynucleotides

3 Recombinant DNA technology is:
  a The modification of mitochondrial RNA
  b Genetic modification
  c The analysis of nuclear DNA
  d RNA sequencing
  e *In vivo* DNA synthesis

4 PCR is the acronym for:
  a Proteinase chain reaction
  b Partition chromatography
  c Polymerase chain reaction
  d Post-chromatic resolution
  e Plasmid core reconstruction

5 Plasmids are:
  a Derived directly from viral DNA
  b Generally accepted to be integral components of chromosomal DNA
  c Cut using non-specific restriction endonucleases
  d Inserted into mitochondrial RNA
  e Carry genes conferring resistance to antibiotics

6 Knockout mice:
  a   Have synthetically designed additional genes
  b   Have genetically engineered muscular enhancement
  c   Have genetically inactivated or removed genes
  d   Do not require stem cell technology
  e   Production require experimentally activated genes

Further reading

Cohen SN, Chang ACY, Boyer HW, Helling RB. Construction of biologically functional bacterial plasmids *in vitro*. *Proc Nat Acad Sci USA* 1973; 70: 3240–4.

Howarth JL, Bok-Lee Y, Uney JB. Using viral vectors as gene transfer tools. *Cell Biol Toxicol* 2010; 26: 1–20.

Kay MA, Glorioso JC, Naldrini L. Viral vectors for gene therapy: the art of turning infectious agents into vehicles of therapeutics. *Nat Med* 2001; 7: 33–40.

Lin JG, Chen WL. Acupuncture analgesia: a review of its mechanisms of action. *Am J Chinese Med* 2008; 36: 635–645.

Relph K, Harrington K, Pandha H. Recent developments and current status of gene therapy using viral vectors in the United Kingdom. *BMJ* 2004; 329: 839–42.

Stein LD. Human genome: End of the beginning. *Nature* 2004; 431: 915–16.

Venter C. Multiple personal genomes await. *Nature* 2010; 464: 676–7.

Yoshida N, Sato M. Plasmid uptake by bacteria: a comparison of methods and efficiencies. *Appl Microbiol* 2009; 83: 791–8.

2

Vaccines

Objectives:

- Be able to give examples of vaccines against diseases, especially those relevant in the UK.
- Know the meanings of the relevant terms mentioned in the mini-glossary.
- Learn the main divisions of immunity.
- Know what is meant by active and passive immunity.
- Be able to outline briefly the mechanisms of action of vaccines given in the text.
- Give an account of modern production methods of vaccines.
- Be familiar with the given procedures and problems facing developers when new vaccines are needed.

Definition of a vaccine

A vaccine is an antigenic preparation derived from a disease-carrying organism that will stimulate the recipient body to develop specific antibodies to it and thereby confer active immunity against the disease.

A brief history

The Chinese have practised various forms of vaccination (or immunisation) for at least 2000 years. Early practitioners noticed that contraction of small-pox conferred immunity against further recurrence, and practised a form of vaccination, also known as variolation. Smallpox, incidentally, was traditionally called variola.

In 1718, Lady Mary Wortley Montague, the wife of the English ambassador to Turkey, noted that the Turks inoculated their children against smallpox and tried unsuccessfully to interest the British scientific establishment in the technique. In 1796, an English vicar and doctor called Edward Jenner injected pus from a cowpox pustule into an incision in an 8-year-old boy's arm, and showed that the boy was subsequently immune to smallpox. His experiment was inspired, at least in part, by farming folklore that milkmaids who caught cowpox never contracted smallpox. Initially rebuffed by The Royal Society, who sent him away to do more work, he gathered further evidence and his contribution was recognised. He coined the word 'vaccine' from the Latin *vacca*, meaning cow, to describe the preparation that he administered. His work was carried on, notably by Louis Pasteur, a nineteenth-century French academic, who most famously introduced the process now known as pasteurisation. He also established the germ theory of disease and built on the work of Jenner in the development of vaccines, notably against rabies, when he used a new invention, the hypodermic syringe, to immunise and save a boy who had been bitten by a rabid dog.

The huge Spanish influenza epidemic of 1918–1919 spurred on efforts for the development of vaccines. Fear of a repetition of more pandemics motivated efforts to develop vaccines directed at many viral infections. A yellow fever vaccine was introduced in 1937 and the successful cultivation of the poliomyelitis virus in the 1940s to 1950s resulted in the polio vaccine. Since then a great many vaccines against diseases have been prepared. The huge problems created by viral and bacterial epidemics among farm animals, both here and abroad, have focused efforts aimed at the rapid production of vaccines against, for example, bluetongue, swine fever and bovine spongiform encephalopathy (BSE). Unfortunately, all attempts to produce a vaccine against HIV have failed (at the time of writing).

Miniglossary

Acquired immunity

Immunity acquired from the development of antibodies in response to an antigen, e.g. after having the disease or after vaccination against it.

Active immunity

The ability of the body's cells to respond to the antigen, i.e. disease, and produce antibodies directed against the disease antigen.

Antibody

Lymphocyte-produced protein directed against and that neutralises a specific antigen.

Antigen

Substance, usually large, e.g. a protein, identified by the organism as foreign, which evokes an immune response.

Attenuated vaccine

Live pathogens that have lost their virulence but are still capable of inducing a protective immune response to the virulent forms of the pathogen, e.g. Sabin polio vaccine. Methods and reagents used include alum precipitation, formaldehyde and heating.

Immunological memory

The capacity of the immune system to respond more rapidly and with an amplified response to a second contact with a specific antigen than to the first contact.

Immunity

Ability of the organism successfully to resist infection through the presence of circulating white blood cells and of tissue-bound and/or circulating antibodies directed against the antigens associated with the disease threatening the body.

Passive immunity

Immunity produced by injection of antibodies produced from the serum of an already immune donor; relatively short-lived immunity.

A nomenclature note: inoculation may be defined as the introduction of any organism where it will survive and grow, whereas vaccination (immunisation) is the administration of an antigenic material, i.e. a vaccine, in order to induce immunity to a given disease. Today, these two are generally used interchangeably. A vaccine may be described as a biologically based preparation, which confers or enhances immunity to a specific disease. In order to understand how vaccines work it is necessary to know some of the basics about immunity.

Immunity

The main divisions of immunity are as follows:

Innate (non-adaptive, non-specific) immunity

- Present from birth
- Includes the body's barriers to pathogens, which are:
    - mechanical barriers, i.e. mucous membranes and skin
    - chemical barriers, e.g. bacteriostatic fatty acids in skin, digestive enzymes and gastric HCl

- the complement system
- phagocytic cells.

Acquired immunity

This is usually immunity to a specific invading organism or a group of related organisms. Acquired immunity may be active or passive.

Active immunity

This occurs when the body's immune system confers immunity against an organism through cellular responses, resulting in the production of antibodies. Active immunity may be acquired through infection with the disease or by vaccination, which confers immunity without the risks associated with the disease symptoms. Active immunity may be one of the following:

- Antibody-mediated immunity, through B cells (B lymphocytes) and plasma cells, which are the progeny of the original B cells. B cells respond to the antigen by producing lymphocytes that produce antibodies to the antigen. B cells are produced and mature in bone marrow. They differ from T cells (see below) because they do not migrate but reside principally in the gastrointestinal tract, spleen and lymph nodes. On activation, they differentiate into antibody-secreting plasma cells.
- Cell-mediated immunity, through T cells (T lymphocytes).

Immunological memory

This consists of two main responses to infection.

The primary response
When infective agents, e.g. viruses or bacteria, invade the body, initially relatively few cells recognise these antigens, with the production of relatively few neutralising antibodies; however, the infection initiates the production of very many memory T and B cells, so that, when the antigen invades a second time, this initiates the secondary response.

The secondary response
When the same antigen re-invades, even years later, this triggers a huge production by the T- and B-memory cells of antibodies highly specific to and of very high affinity for the antigen, which is rapidly neutralised.

Passive immunity

This is generally a short-lived immunity (weeks or months) to a particular pathogen through the introduction of antibodies originally generated in an immune individual. Passive immunity is naturally transferred across the placenta. The protection conferred through cross-placental passive immunisation differs with the pathogen, e.g. protection of the fetus from measles is greater than that from polio and whooping cough, also known as pertussis, because the latter is caused by the bacterium *Bordetella pertussis*. (Infection, incidentally, that triggers *active* immunisation may offer life-long protection.)

Mechanism of action of vaccines

Vaccines confer protection against a specific disease by:

- induction of active immunity
- conferring immunological memory.

Vaccines are generally administered in divided doses, separated by intervals, which (1) permit the immune system to respond by producing antigen-specific B cells, IgM and plasma cells, which produce IgG, and (2) to amplify the immune system's response to subsequent doses of vaccine.

Production of vaccines

This aspect of vaccine science has assumed huge importance through fears of widespread influenza epidemics or pandemics that could result if, for example, the avian H5N1 influenza virus mutates and become infective in humans when air borne. There is now intense focus on the mass production and rapid distribution of vaccines.

Historically, the report of the successful growth of poliomyelitis virus in human embryonic tissue by Weller, Robbins and Enders in 1949 was the impetus for the successful clinical development by Salk and his colleagues of a vaccine against poliomyelitis, and many bacterial and viral infections can now be prevented by vaccination.

Modern production methods

The ideal method for vaccine production should include these qualities:

- rapid production, especially in times of pandemic threat
- economical
- inherently safe
- high affinity for the target
- low antigenicity for the host body
- stable
- production of a vaccine with high immunogenicity.

Methods

- Using fertilised chicken eggs
- Using tissue or cell culture

- Using transgenic plants
- Using recombinant DNA technology.

Although these headings are represented separately, modern methods often involve more than one, e.g. recombinant DNA technology is heavily relied on in the production of transgenic plants in order to produce variants that will express the antigen of interest.

Using fertilised chicken eggs

The virus, e.g. a strain of the influenza virus, is injected into a fertilised egg, usually about 11 days after fertilisation. The virus infects the embryo and multiplies. After a predetermined number of days, the eggs are opened by machine and the virus is harvested, purified, inactivated (attenuated) by chemical means and processed into a clinically usable product.

The process has some disadvantages in that it is laborious and it can take up to 6 months or more to prepare the vaccine in bulk. One egg may yield only two doses of vaccine and delays due to egg production are a time-limiting factor. Clearly this method might not meet the demand in the event of an unexpected pandemic of, for example, influenza.

There may also be an adverse reaction in recipients who are allergic to eggs. This has been an issue with the MMR (measles, mumps and rubella) and polio vaccine in egg-sensitive children, who in the past may not have been vaccinated, but it is now generally considered more important to confer protection. Other problems with eggs include the possible presence of other viral strains and antibiotics, and the possibility that other variant species of virus antigenically distinct from the virus being targeted may be present.

Using tissue or cell culture

The ideal cell line should include these properties:

- propagate the virus in abundance rapidly and efficiently
- should be adaptable to different strains of the virus, especially and now, topically, to the influenza virus
- should be amenable to propagation in synthetic media, free if possible from large animal-derived molecules, e.g. proteins
- should be adaptable for large-scale production
- licensing requirements for the cell line should not pose problems.

The media may be synthetic or serum based.

This was the method originally used by Enders and his colleagues in their pioneering work with poliomyelitis virus grown on human foreskin tissue.

The tissue, e.g. mammalian kidney cells, is infected with the virus and the cells and virus both multiply in number. The virus is harvested from the cell or tissue culture, and purified and inactivated, e.g. the rabies virus may be inactivated using ethyleneimine. This, too, is a relatively long process due to the time taken, not only for tissue or cell culture, but also during the purification, standardisation and validation procedures. Advantages over egg use include the elimination of possible allergy issues and the delays associated with egg production.

Using transgenic plants

Plants are now viable alternatives for consideration as media for vaccine production thanks to the advances in molecular biology. It is possible to genetically engineer plants that will express bacterial and viral antigens. Some that have been successfully produced include the transformation of tobacco plants to induce them to express the *Streptococcus mutans* surface protein antigen A and the F1 and LcrV antigens of *Yersinia pestis* (cause of the plague). This approach is interesting but still very much in the developmental stage at the time of writing. It will undoubtedly raise concerns among population groups who oppose any form of genetic engineering in crops.

Enhancement of immunogenicity

Adjuvant chemicals are added to vaccines to enhance the vaccine's ability to elicit a powerful cellular immune response after administration. Earlier adjuvants included, for example, tapioca, bread and alum. Today, vaccine developers are exploring other adjuvants, e.g. the use of oil-in-water emulsions and highly specific nucleotide sequences of bacterial DNA, c.g. CpG2 oligodeoxynucleotides. CpG2 is a synapse-specific protein in the brain that regulates the endocytosis of glutamate receptors and is important in the mechanisms underlying postsynaptic plasticity.

Paradigm of a coordinated response to the threat of an influenza pandemic

The rate of spread of the Spanish flu and the recent scare over a possible pandemic of H5N1 influenza provide an example of the problems facing those who need rapid identification of the infective agent, and the large-scale production and distribution of an effective vaccine to be directed against just such an organism. This requires globally coordinated collection of both clinical and epidemiological data, the practical steps in identification and isolation of the infective agent and, ideally, the rapid mass production and distribution of an effective vaccine. This is the remit of the World Health

Organization (WHO), working in coordination with national influenza agencies, laboratories and vaccine manufacturers. The most serious obstacle, arguably, is the time taken to develop a vaccine, which in the case of influenza could, given the present technical status, involve several months or more than 1 year. The sequence of steps given below is a highly summarised account of a painfully long, laborious and painstaking process that requires extensive global coordination and cooperation.

Continuous, global clinical surveillance of influenza outbreaks is essential. If there is an outbreak, e.g. of flu, specimens have to be collected, the virus identified and biochemically analysed, including complete genetic sequencing. This alone may take several weeks. Simultaneously it is necessary to find out if previously prepared vaccines will neutralise the new virus. These procedures require extensive collaboration and represent a lengthy process, involving week or even months.

The new virus has to be grown, most probably, in eggs or in MDCK (Madin–Darby canine kidney) cells. Next, the virus is injected into animals, e.g. ferrets, in order to generate antibodies to the virus. Ferrets are notoriously susceptible to flu viruses, and must be cleared of viral infections before being deliberately infected with the virus of interest. In addition, infected ferrets have to be securely isolated after infection. This process could take another month. The ferret antisera then have to be analysed for antigenicity and genetic sequencing, which involves anything from 1 week to 1 month. If the antiserum is found to be effective against the virus of interest, it then has to be manufactured in bulk and distributed. The whole process could take 6 months to a year.

Some examples of specific vaccines

Clearly this is a highly selective list of vaccines; readers are referred to the *BNF* and *Immunisation against Infectious Diseases* (Salisbury et al. 2008) for more comprehensive lists.

Anthrax vaccine

Anthrax is an acute infectious disease in farm animals caused by *Bacillus anthracis* and is transmitted by spores in, for example, animal hair, bones or hides, and can survive for long periods in the soil. Symptoms depend on the route of infection and may include cutaneous lesions, influenza-like symptoms, or abdominal pain and diarrhoea. The incidence in humans is relatively rare and confined mainly to farm workers. The vaccine is a sterile filtrate of alum-precipitated anthrax antigen (Sterne strain of the bacillus) in a solution for injection containing thiomersal as preservative.

Indications and dosage

Anthrax immunisation is indicated for laboratory staff working with the bacillus, those who work with infected animals and those who handle infected products from abroad. The dosage regimen is an initial course of three intramuscular injections, each 3 weeks apart, followed by a single dose 6 months later and a follow-up booster dose once yearly. Each dose should preferentially be given at a site distant from the one before, and at least 2.5–3.0 cm apart. The vaccine should not be given to patients severely ill with anthrax unless urgent, because it may erroneously be blamed for any symptoms and not used further. Patients with only minor symptoms should be considered for vaccination. Specialist advice should always be sought. In the UK, all cases of anthrax have to be reported

Contraindications

Few: history of anaphylactic response to a previous dose of anthrax vaccine or to any of the ingredients of the vaccine.

Adverse effects reported after injection

These include: swelling, pain and redness as common reactions at the site of injection; urticaria, mild temperature and symptoms of flu. Reactions considered serious should be reported (in the UK) via the Yellow Card scheme.

Cholera vaccine

Cholera is caused by *Vibrio cholerae*, a Gram-negative bacterium. The bacterium multiplies rapidly after infection and symptoms may appear within hours of infection. The symptoms are a sudden onset of copious liquid stools, usually accompanied by severe abdominal pain. The loss of water and electrolytes may be life threatening if left untreated. These require rapid replacement. The bacterium generates an endotoxin locally that is responsible for the diarrhoea. The source is often contaminated seafood, especially shellfish, or contaminated drinking water. Infective subgroups or biotypes of cholera exist, e.g. the so-called El Tor or classic, which is further subdivided into biotypes, the most predominant being a subtype, called Ogawa.

In the UK, the only vaccine currently available is Dukoral, for oral administration, consisting of an aqueous suspension in buffer of formaldehyde + heat-inactivated Inaba and Ogawa strains of *Vibrio cholerae*, together with recombinant cholera toxin B. The Inaba strains include the El Tor subtype. Before administration, this is diluted with a freshly prepared solution of effervescent sodium bicarbonate granules in water, and the dosage adjusted by dilution of the vaccine according to age. The patients should be nil by mouth 1 hour before and after administration of the vaccine. The *BNF* recommends that, for adults and children aged >6 years, the dose should be repeated 1–6 weeks after the first dose; for children aged 2–6 years there should be three doses, each separated by 1–6 weeks. The second dose should not be given after more than 6 weeks, in which case the primary course should be started again (see *BNF* and Salisbury *et al.* 2008 for more dosage details). Vaccination should not, however, be assumed to confer complete protection to those who visit countries in which cholera is endemic, and sensible, informed attitudes to diet and hygiene should be adopted. In the UK, cholera is a notifiable disease.

Contraindications

These include a previous anaphylactic reaction to a dose of cholera vaccine, or to any of the ingredients used, notably formaldehyde. The vaccine should not be used in patients acutely ill with gastrointestinal problems.

Hepatitis B vaccine

Hepatitis B is caused through infection with the hepatitis B virus. This is a DNA virus that targets and replicates primarily in liver hepatocytes, causing inflammation. It is endemic in parts of Africa and Asia and periodic epidemics occur. Infections may be self-limiting, i.e. be cleared by the body, or become chronic. In some cases, the infection may be completely asymptomatic. After infection, there is an incubation period that may last from about 10 weeks to 5 months. Symptoms initially are of general malaise, with nausea, vomiting, mild pyrexia, loss of appetite, skin itchiness and discoloured urine, which darkens. Faeces become noticeably lighter in colour. Jaundice develops. In most cases, symptoms lessen and after 2 or 3 weeks they disappear altogether. In some cases, the liver rapidly becomes severely damaged (fulminant hepatic failure), which may prove fatal. If infection is diagnosed, patients are encouraged to abstain from alcohol, which could exacerbate any cirrhosis.

Diagnosis is through blood tests for viral antigens, notably the hepatitis B surface antigen (HBsAg), and for host-produced antibodies to the virus, e.g. anti-HBc IgM (antibody to the hepatitis B core antigen). If HBsAg persists in serum for 6 months or longer then this is considered to be chronic infection with hepatitis B, and these people are the so-called 'carriers' of hepatitis B.

Transmission of hepatitis B is through introduction of the virus via parenteral routes, e.g. shared needles, through vaginal or anal sexual intercourse, or through perinatal transmission to the newborn child from the mother.

High-risk groups among the population include those who misuse drugs that require injection, those with whom they are intimate and their children. Others at risk include those who frequently change their sexual partners (see the *BNF* for a more comprehensive list of high-risk individuals). In the UK, there is now minimal risk of infection through transfusion as donated blood is screened for hepatitis B, and blood products are routinely treated to inactivate viruses.

Hepatitis B vaccine consists of inactivated HBsAg adsorbed onto aluminium hydroxide or phosphate adjuvants for intramuscular injection into the anterolateral thigh or upper arm. The buttocks are avoided due to inefficient absorption of the vaccine. The vaccines do not possess the infective agent and are unable to cause hepatitis B infection. Dosage regimens vary among the different proprietary preparations, but, in general terms, after the initial injection, further single doses are administered each month for 3 or 4 months. Dosage regimens vary among the different preparations and the reader is referred to the *BNF* for further information about this. Not all patients respond well in terms of protection against hepatitis B. Factors known to impair vaccination efficiency include smoking, obesity, alcohol in excess and those aged >40 years.

MMR vaccination

The MMR vaccination is a mixture of attenuated, live and freeze-dried preparations of measles, mumps and rubella viruses. Measles is caused by a paramyxovirus, which is an airborne virus. These target, predominantly, the respiratory system and cause, for example, mumps and measles (*myxo* is Greek for mucus). Measles is extremely infectious and may be transmitted by aerosol and even through cohabitation. Contagion extends from the first appearance of symptoms through to 3–5 days after the first appearance of the rash.

Mumps is caused by another paramyxovirus, which is also an airborne virus. It is less contagious than measles, and infection results from relatively close contact. It has a long incubation period, the time from initial infection to appearance of symptoms being as long as 3 weeks. Initial symptoms, typically, are a few days of physical discomfort with pyrexia, followed by swelling of the parotid salivary glands, where the virus is concentrated. Swellings may persist for about a week or more.

The rubella virus causes German measles. It occurs most commonly in children but can infect at any age. Rubella is transmitted both by air and through direct contact. In most cases the disease is mild, but in pregnant women, especially within the first 10 weeks of pregnancy, is highly dangerous to the fetus, which may be born with serious deformities.

Symptoms, typically, include swollen glands at the back of the neck and behind the ears. Symptoms of a cold, including a sore throat and cough, may occur, or it may be asymptomatic. After about 7 days a rash may appear on the face and spread to other parts of the body. The rash is usually gone after about 5 days. Adults may experience joint pains.

The MMR vaccine is usually in two doses to children before their entry into primary school. In the UK, the first dose is given at 13 months, and the second dose between 3 and 5 years of age, before the children enter primary school.

Contraindications to the MMR include pregnancy (see above), patients whose immune systems are weakened through, for example, HIV infection, or if a previous live vaccine has been given within the preceding 4 weeks.

An ethical perspective

It is not uncommon to meet parents who wish to exert their right to refuse vaccination on the part of their children. Some believe in unproven alternative approaches to disease prevention, e.g. homoeopathy; others justify their decisions by feeling uncomfortable about injecting their children against an infective agent that they are unlikely to contract in their lifetime, or worrying that there may be hidden side effects or complications from the vaccine that have not been discovered yet.

An example of the fragile equilibrium between perceived benefits and risks of vaccines was the recent MMR scare. Measles vaccination started in 1968, and a steady decrease in the incidence of measles was observed. In the 1990s when vaccine uptake was very high (>92%) measles incidence and associated mortality were very low.

In 1998 a team of London researchers suggested a possible link between the MMR vaccine and both autism and some gastrointestinal problems. Despite several subsequent and larger studies negating this finding, public hysteria ensued and there was a significant fall in the uptake of MMR vaccination between 1998 and 2001 (<79% uptake). Despite several education programmes, uptake has still not returned to pre-1998 levels (currently 84%), and there has been an increase in the incidence of measles notification over several years. It is thought that MMR uptake of 90% is needed to maintain herd immunity and prevent endemic spread.

There are times when it is difficult as a clinician to accept the right of patients, or patients' guardians, to decline immunisation. This is particularly the case when one is aware that their interpretation of the evidence base is incorrect. However, it is important to remember that all patients have the autonomy to make their own decisions, and that the role of the clinician is to give balanced information and let the patient decide.

Further information on immunisation is given in the *BNF*.

Multiple choice questions

For each question, five options are provided and only one is correct.

1 A vaccine is:
   a   An antigenic preparation derived from a disease-free organism that provides protection against disease
   b   An injection that stimulates the body to develop non-specific antibodies
   c   Administered only by injection
   d   Also termed 'an inoculation'
   e   In need of a recipient immune system with immunological memory resources

2 Immunological memory is:
   a   The capacity of the immune system to respond more rapidly to a second challenge by an antibody
   b   The property of thymus cells to store B cells
   c   The ability of the immune system to respond more rapidly and with an amplified response to a second contact with an antigen
   d   Immunity produced by genetic modification of T lymphocytes
   e   A property of retroviruses

3 Inoculation is:
   a   The introduction of an antigenic substance by intramuscular injection
   b   Application of an antigenic substance to the ear
   c   Induction of ophthalmic antibodies
   d   Introduction of an organism where it will survive and grow
   e   Conferring immunity after exposure to a foreign antigen

4 Innate immunity:
   a   Is present from birth
   b   Is an adaptive, highly specific immunity
   c   Is provided by maternal interleukins
   d   Is threatened by the complement system
   e   Develops early during fetal development

5 Active immunity:
   a   May be acquired through production by the host immune system of specific antigens
   b   Is inhibited by viral DNA
   c   May be conferred through antibody production
   d   Is cell mediated through B-lymphocyte activation
   e   Results from B-cell production of erythrocytes

6 Passive immunity:
  a   Is produced by injection of antibodies produced from the serum of an already immune donor
  b   Is generally a long-lived immunity
  c   Is not transferred across the placenta
  d   Is infectious
  e   Is an adverse effect of immunisation

7 Vaccines confer protection against disease by:
  a   Inhibiting natural immunity
  b   Promoting production of antigen-specific B cells, IgM and plasma cells
  c   Inhibiting plasma cell production
  d   Blocking cytokine production
  e   Limiting the immune response to subsequent challenge by the antigen

8 Vaccines are produced using:
  a   Fertilised chicken eggs
  b   Cultured murine liver
  c   Deactivated virus supernatant
  d   Lymph nodes
  e   Salmon fibroblasts

9 Properties of the ideal cell or tissue culture:
  a   Low protein concentration
  b   High specificity for a single viral strain
  c   Intolerant to synthetic chemicals
  d   Rigid and tightly controlled criteria for licensing before use
  e   Better suited to small batch technology

10 Vaccine immunogenicity is enhanced by:
  a   Avoiding adjuvants
  b   Using non-specific nucleotide sequences of bacterial DNA
  c   Raising the concentration of carbohydrates
  d   The use of oil-in-water emulsions
  e   Sterilising the vaccine at high temperatures

11 Specific vaccines:
  a   Anthrax vaccine should not be given to patients ill with anthrax unless urgent
  b   Cholera is caused by *Vibrio cholerae*, a Gram-positive bacterium
  c   Hepatitis B is transmitted orally
  d   MMR vaccine is a mixture of measles, mumps and rabies vaccines
  e   Rubella virus causes mumps

References

Salisbury D, Ramsay M, Noakes K, eds. *Immunisation against Infectious Disease*. London: The Stationery Office, 2006.

Weller TH, Robbins FC, Enders JF. Cultivation of poliomyelitis virus in cultures of human foreskin and embryonic tissues. *Proc Soc Expl Biol* 1949; 72: 153–5.

Further reading

Balsano C. Recent advances in antiviral agents: established and innovative therapies for viral hepatitis. *Mini Rev Med Chem* 2008; 8: 307–18.

Collins SA, Guinn BA, Harrison PT, Scallon MF, O'Sullivan GC, Tangney M. Viral vectors in cancer immunotherapy: which vector for which strategy? *Curr Gene Ther* 2008; 8: 66–78.

Cools N, Ponsaerts P, Van Tendeloo VF, Berneman ZN. Regulatory T cells and human disease. *Clin Dev Immunol* 2007; 8915.

Cottrell JR, Borok E, Horvath TL, Nedivi E. CPG2: a brain- and synapse-specific protein that regulates the endocytosis of glutamate receptors. *Neuron* 2004; 44: 677–90.

Floss MF, Falkenburg D, Conrad U. Production of vaccines and therapeutic antibodies for veterinary applications in transgenic plants: an overview. *Transgenic Res* 2007; 16: 315–32.

Hoft DF. Tuberculosis vaccine development: goals, immunological design, and evaluation. *Lancet* 2008; 372: 164–75.

Lico C, Chen Q, Santi L. Viral vectors for production of recombinant proteins in plants. *J Cell Physiol* 2008; 216: 366–77.

Morris SK, Moss WJ, Halsey N. *Haemophilus influenzae* type b conjugate vaccine use and effectiveness. *Lancet Infect Dis* 2008; 8: 435–43.

Orenstein WA, Schaffner W. Lessons learned: role of influenza vaccine production, distribution, supply, and demand – what it means for the provider. *Am J Med* 2008; 121(7 suppl 2): S22–S77.

Tůve O, Cravens PD, Eager TN. DNA-based vaccines: the future of multiple sclerosis therapy? *Expert Rev Neurother* 2008; 8: 351–60.

3

Hormone-related drugs

Objectives:

- Be able to outline the fundamentals of the brain–pituitary–endocrine–organ axis.
- Know the anatomical location of the thyroid gland and of its major hormonal secretions, as well as the basic cellular processes of the thyroid cell.
- Be ready to answer questions on the actions of the thyroid hormones and the control of their release.
- Be able to give examples of the clinical use of the thyroid hormones.
- Name the three zones of the adrenal cortex and the major endocrine hormones secreted by each zone.
- Be familiar with the endocrine control of adrenal steroid release.
- Know the nature of the adrenal medullary hormones, their mechanism of action, endocrine actions and uses.
- Know the nature and uses of the sex hormones and also Trastuzumab.
- Be ready to answer questions on insulin, its receptor, mechanism of action and uses.
- Know something of the nature, actions, mechanism of actions and uses of growth hormone.
- Know what is meant by the incretins and their location, actions and potential use for diabetes.

Knowledge of hormone identity and mechanism of action has generated a huge battery of important drugs that either mimic or block the actions of endogenous hormones, or promote or inhibit hormone synthesis and release. Many of these medicinally used compounds include naturally occurring substances, e.g. estradiol, insulin, thyroxine, luteinising hormone-releasing hormone (LHRH) and cortisol. Several are now synthesised. Examples appear in this chapter, which is organised in terms of the hormonal systems from which the drugs are derived.

The elucidation of the role of the brain–pituitary axis in the control of hormone production and release by the endocrine glands has resulted in drugs such as the oral contraceptives, which have transformed society, and also some very useful diagnostic tests in order to localise a lesion in the brain–pituitary–target organ axis. An unfortunate example of a negative impact of knowledge about hormone action is the widespread use of anabolic steroids to enhance physical performance in competitive sport. On a more positive note, millions of patients have benefited from the availability of hormones and their antagonists for the treatment of, for example, malignant diseases, diabetes, thyroid disorders, growth problems and infertility.

Brief history

The existence of the so-called 'ductless' glands preoccupied scientists from as early as the 1830s. The visible manifestations of thyroid disorders stimulated much early work, and in the 1890s George Murray successfully treated myxoedema with thyroid extracts. The connection between the pancreas and diabetes was recognised in the mid-1800s, when pancreatic extracts were given orally (and unsuccessfully) to treat sugar diabetes. The word 'hormone' was derived by Ernest Henry Starling from the Greek word ὁρμή – 'to set in motion' or 'arouse' – when he and William Bayliss reported their discovery of secretin in 1902. Their experiment illustrates the ingenuity of early experiments by pharmacologists with relatively few research tools. They severed the nervous innervation between the pancreas and duodenum, and found that, in the absence of nervous innervation between two organs, the pancreas nevertheless released a hormone into the circulation in order to promote duodenal digestive secretions after food intake.

In the 1920s, Frederick Banting, Charles Best and John McLeod in Toronto successfully treated a child with diabetes using an injectable extract from dog pancreas, which resulted in the discovery of insulin. From the 1930s onwards, the rate of discovery of the steroid hormones accelerated, and the ovaries, adrenals and testes yielded the adrenocortical and reproductive steroid hormones, which became available to the medical profession. The introduction of the glucocorticoids for the treatment of rheumatoid arthritis produced dramatic improvements when initially administered, and were hailed as a great medical discovery and virtually a cure until the serious adverse effects of prolonged use of synthetic glucocorticoids became apparent.

During the 1940s and 1950s, Geoffrey Harris, who is considered by many to be the founding father of neuroendocrinology, provided experimental evidence for the existence of a portal blood system between the hypothalamus and the anterior pituitary gland. Previous workers had suspected the link, but it was Harris, using India ink, who visualised it. This was the impetus that resulted in the identification of the hypothalamic–anterior pituitary hormonal systems that mediate the feedback effects of hormones, and in the development of drugs to treat, for example, thyroid and adrenocortical problems. Work carried out by the American scientist Dr Gregory Pincus and his associates resulted in the introduction of oral contraceptives in the early 1960s, and in 1977 Rosalyn Yalow, Roger Guillemin and Andrew Schally shared the Nobel Prize for Medicine for the elucidation of the structure of LHRH (a gonadotrophin-releasing hormone or GnRH).

Advances in biotechnology have fed into drug development, and there is now a far more powerful and sophisticated approach to the development of hormone-related disease treatment. The realisation of the once-mythical 'magic bullet' has become a more credible aim with the tools provided by molecular biology.

Thyroid hormones

The thyroid gland is situated in the neck close to the trachea (Figure 3.1).

The thyroid secretes the hormones thyroxine (T_4) and triiodothyronine (T_3) from the thyroid follicle cell. These hormones travel in the bloodstream largely bound to a specific thyroid-binding globulin (TBG). As is the case for many hormones, it is the free, unbound hormone that is available to the tissues. T_3 is more powerful than T_4, and most tissues convert T_4 to T_3. These hormones regulate the metabolic rate by:

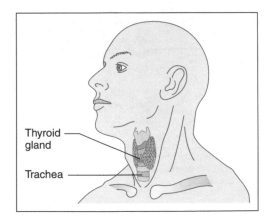

Thyroid gland

Trachea

Figure 3.1 Position of the thyroid gland in the neck.

- generating sufficient energy to maintain normal body temperature through ATP synthesis and mitochondrial oxygen consumption
- enhancing absorption of glucose in the gastrointestinal tract
- limiting insulin action by speeding its rate of breakdown
- potentiating glycogen $\Rightarrow$ glucose in liver (glycogenolysis) and by action of adrenaline
- reducing plasma cholesterol
- stimulating vitamin A synthesis.

Control of thyroid hormone synthesis and release

Thyroid hormone synthesis and release are controlled by the hypothalamic–pituitary gland axis through a negative feedback system (Figure 3.2). Clearly, under- or oversecretion of thyroid hormones will disturb the negative feedback system, resulting in hypo- or hyperthyroidism; knowledge of the system and armed with the tools for measuring T_3, T_4, thyroid-stimulating hormone (TSH) and thyrotrophin-releasing hormone (TRH), we are able to test it.

The hypothalamic–anterior pituitary axis also controls the synthesis and release of the adrenocortical and gonadal hormones (see later). The thyroid hormones are synthesised in and released from the thyroid follicle cell (Figure 3.3)

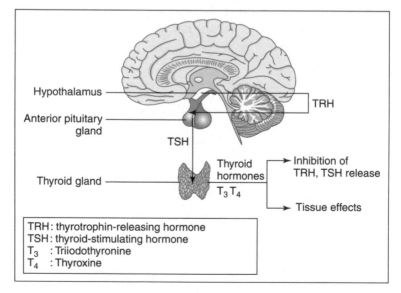

Figure 3.2 Negative feedback control of thyroid hormone release.

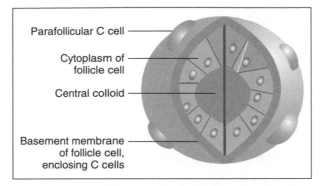

Figure 3.3 Thyroid follicle cells surrounding the central colloid circulate in the bloodstream; in the brain and anterior pituitary gland they inhibit the release of thyrotrophin-releasing hormone (TRH) and thyroxine-releasing hormone, respectively. Pathological or pharmacological intervention may upset the regulatory system and result in hypo- or hyperthyroidism.

Thyroid hormone synthesis and release (Figure 3.4)

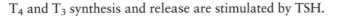

T_4 and T_3 synthesis and release are stimulated by TSH.

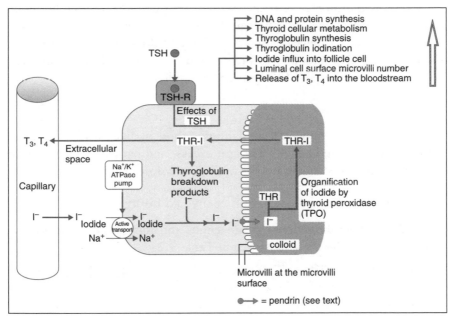

Figure 3.4 Diagrammatic thyroid follicle cell and luminal colloid: effects of thyroid-stimulating hormone (TSH).

Mechanism of action of thyroid hormones

Thyroid hormones effect their actions through binding to: (1) intranuclear receptor proteins that alter transcription (see also Adrenal hormones and The sex hormones for mechanism of action of steroid hormones); (2) mitochondrial receptor proteins; and (3) possibly specific cell membrane proteins in some tissues. At least three different isoforms of thyroid hormone receptors have been described, namely α_1, β_1 and β_2. Thyroid hormones bind to their receptors with high affinity and specificity; mutations of thyroid receptors have been reported, which bind the hormone poorly, and that could explain reported cases of thyroid hormone resistance.

Clinical uses of thyroid hormones

Hypothyroidism is usually treated using thyroxine orally in tablet form.

Thyroxine is prescribed as levothyroxine (thyroxine) sodium, and may be prescribed as 25, 50 or 100 µg tablets, or as an oral solution. Liothyranine(L-triiodothyronine) is usually prescribed orally in doses from 10 µg daily to a maximum of 60 µg daily in two to three divided doses.

Before giving thyroxine, it is important to rule out hypopituitarism with hypoadrenal function. This is because thyroxine will speed up adrenal steroid metabolism, which in these patients could precipitate a hypoadrenal crisis.

Hyperthyroidism may be treated with drugs that block thyroid hormone synthesis, or by surgery or radiological methods. The most commonly used drug is probably carbimazole. Iodine or iodide salts may be prescribed for thyrotoxicosis. The best-known preparation is probably Lugol's solution, containing 5% iodine and 10% potassium iodide in purified water.

Thyrotoxicosis

Although thyroid hormones occur naturally, these, unlike the case for many other hormones, can be highly toxic in excess, and patients taking thyroid hormones need to be monitored for signs of overdose (Table 3.1).

Effects of other drugs on secretion of thyroid hormones

Many drugs affect the actions of endogenous and administered thyroid hormones and examples are summarised in Table 3.2.

Table 3.1 Signs of thyroid hormone overdosage				
Cardiovascular	**Nervous system**	**Gastrointestinal tract**	**Hair, skin**	**Musculoskeletal**
Congestive heart failure Exacerbation of angina Tachycardia	Anxiety Exophthalmos[a] Insomnia Irritability and short temper Nervous	Diarrhoea Increased appetite Thirst	Loss and thinning of hair Increased sweating Intolerance to heat	Osteoporosis Proximal muscle weakness[b] Exaggerated deep tendon reflexes

[a] Lid retraction and bulging eyeball.
[b] Weakness at or near the point of insertion of muscle (or tendon).

Table 3.2 Effects of some drugs on thyroid hormone activity

Drug	Effects on thyroid activity
Aluminium hydroxide, ferrous sulphate	Decrease absorption (higher dose of T_4 needed)
Lithium	Inhibits thyroid hormone secretion
Carbamazepine, phenytoin	Increase liver metabolism of T_4, T_3
β Blockers, glucocorticoids	Impair conversion of T_4 to T_3
NSAIDs and salicylates	Impair binding of T_3 and T_4 to TBG, thus potentiate their action

T_3, triiodothyronine; T_4, thyroxine; TBG, thyroid-binding globulin.

Case history: hypothyroidism

Bernadette, a 48-year-old woman, went to see her general practitioner apologising for fear of wasting his time. Her symptoms were diffuse and had been developing over many months. She had gained weight, and noticed thinning and coarsening of her hair. Menstruation had become a little heavier than before, although her cycle remained regular. Her main complaint was that she was very tired all the time, and that she had become snappy and irritable with her family. She had been talking to friends, who had advised seeing the doctor, wondering whether she might be approaching the menopause.

Examination by the doctor confirmed the weight gain but this was otherwise unremarkable. Routine blood investigations were organised and confirmed hypothyroidism (T_4: TSH 32.4), ruling out anaemia and the climacteric, which had been raised as other possibilities. The high titre of thyroid peroxidase antibodies confirmed autoimmune hypothyroidism and she was started on thyroid replacement therapy with thyroxine 50 μg once daily. After 8 weeks the dose was increased to 75 μg once daily when the thyroid function tests were repeated and the TSH was still raised (6.4). The subsequent tests confirmed good control and, more importantly, Bernadette was feeling significantly better. She will need annual thyroid function tests and is aware that her treatment will be life-long.

Adrenal hormones

The adrenal glands are situated above the kidneys and are structurally and functionally differentiated into the outer cortex, which secretes the adrenal corticosteroids, and the inner medulla, which secretes the catecholamines adrenaline (epinephrine) and noradrenaline (norepinephrine).

The adrenal cortex

Structurally, the adrenal cortex is further differentiated structurally into: (1) an outer zona glomerulosa, which elaborates the mineralocorticoids aldosterone, and the weaker deoxycorticosterone; (2) a relatively thick middle zone, the zona fasciculata, which elaborates the corticosteroids, also called glucocorticoids, principally cortisol in humans, and the androgens androstenedione, 17α-hydroxyprogesterone and dehydroepiandrosterone sulphate (DHAS); and (3) an inner layer, the zona reticularis, which also secretes corticosteroids and androgens.

Biosynthesis of the adrenal steroids

Elucidation of the biosynthetic pathways of the adrenal steroids (Figure 3.5) paved the way for a greater understanding of problems produced by conditions such as congenital adrenal hyperplasia and Cushing's and Addison's diseases, and provided the rationale for their treatment with steroids and inhibitors of steroidogenesis.

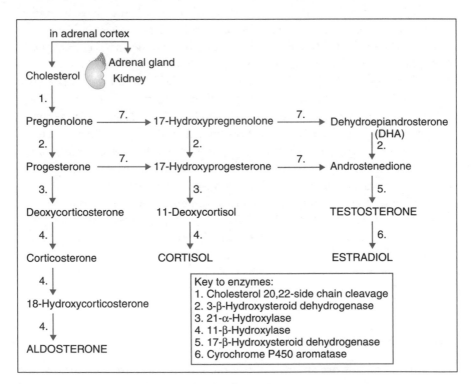

Figure 3.5   Adrenal steroidogenic pathways.

Control of cortisol release (Figure 3.6)

The hypothalamus releases corticotrophin-releasing hormone (CRH) into the anterior pituitary portal system. CRH acts on anterior pituitary adrenocorti-cotrophin-releasing cells, which release adrenocorticotrophin (ACTH) into the general circulation. ACTH stimulates cortisol release from the adrenal cortex. Circulating cortisol limits its own release through a negative feedback action on CRH-producing cells in the hypothalamus and on ACTH-producing cells in the anterior pituitary gland.

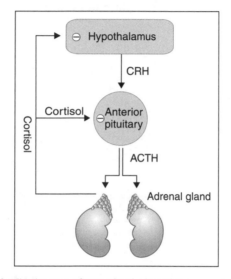

Figure 3.6 Negative feedback action of cortisol in the hypothalamus and anterior pituitary gland – a basis for diagnosis and therapy.

The identification of this system and the availability of CRH, ACTH and cortisol, together with assays of the three substances, enable the clinician to test the integrity of the system.

Examples of the clinical uses of these natural hormone substances are the diagnostic tests for Cushing's disease, including the measurement of urinary free cortisol, and the CRH test followed by ACTH measurement to explore the possibility of, for example, an ectopic ACTH-secreting tumour. Chemical knowledge of the hypothalamic, anterior pituitary and adrenal hormones made possible the development of ACTH analogues and of a battery of glucocorticoids.

Mechanism of action of the adrenal steroids

Aldosterone and cortisol, similar to other steroid hormones, act mainly through intracellular receptor proteins (see Figure 3.6).

The adrenal medulla

The adrenal medulla synthesises and releases the catecholamines, mainly adrenaline, and, to a lesser extent, noradrenaline. Adrenaline is the hormone of 'fight or flight' and noradrenaline is the principal neurotransmitter of the adrenergic division of the autonomic nervous system.

The catecholamines

Adrenaline and noradrenaline are secreted from the adrenal medulla. The biosynthesis of the two catecholamines is shown in Figure 3.7.

Mechanism of action of adrenaline and noradrenaline

Adrenaline and noradrenaline bind to G (guanine)-protein-coupled adrenoceptors on the cell membrane. A brief summary of actions and receptors mediating these is given in Figure 3.8.

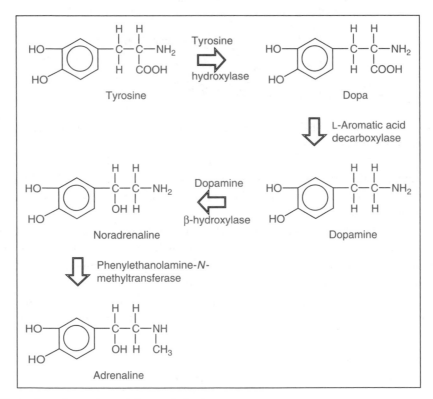

Figure 3.7 Biosynthesis of the catecholamines.

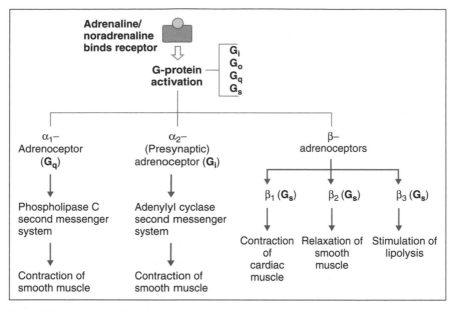

Figure 3.8 Summary of adrenoceptor action.

Clinical uses of adrenaline

- Anaphylactic shock:
    - intramuscular adrenaline 1 mg/mL with close monitoring of blood pressure, respiratory function and pulse rate; depending on these parameters, further doses may be necessary
    - slow intravenous injection of 50 μg adrenaline if there is a poor response to intramuscular administration (see the *BNF* for more details)
- Cardiopulmonary resuscitation:
    - intravenous injection via a central line of 1 mg adrenaline (10 mL of a 100 μg/mL solution of adrenaline); a central line is a catheter that provides venous access via, for example, the right atrium or the superior vena cava
    - alternatively, a peripheral intravenous route may be used provided that there is adequate flushing after the dose with 20 mL sterile saline.

Glaucoma

Glaucoma is caused by closure of the duct of Schlemm at the angle between the cornea and iris where drainage of the aqueous humour usually occurs. This raises the intraocular pressure, which if left untreated invariably results in blindness. Treatment includes the use of a topical prostaglandin analogue, e.g. travoprost, a β blocker, e.g. betaxolol, the carbonic anhydrase inhibitor diuretic acetazolamide, an anticholinesterase, typically pilocarpine, and adrenaline, which promotes drainage and slowing the rate of production of aqueous humour.

Local anaesthesia

Adrenaline is used as an adjunct to local anaesthetics, because it causes local vasoconstriction at the site of injection, thereby slowing drainage of the local anaesthetic.

Croup

This is an acute inflammation of the respiratory tract, which occurs most commonly between 6 months and 3 years of age. Mild croup often resolves spontaneously, but severe cases may require intubation and oral or parenteral corticosteroids. Uncontrolled croup may require nebulised adrenaline under close supervision.

The sex hormones

These include:

- oestrogens
- progesterone
- androgens.

The sex hormones, particularly in the female, do not act in isolation but together in order to maintain fertility and reproductive success. In the male, the testes are the primary source of androgens, and in the female the ovaries are the primary source of oestrogens, mainly estradiol and progesterone. The menstrual cycle is a tightly and highly synchronised sequence of estradiol and progesterone release from the ovary and corpus luteum, respectively, which ensures the optimal intrauterine conditions for ovum release, fertilisation and implantation.

Mechanism of action of sex hormones

Sex hormones, similar to the adrenal steroids, act mainly through intracellular receptor proteins, which bind the hormones selectively, and with high binding affinity (Figure 3.9).

The lipophilic sex hormones, which are uncharged, pass easily through the cell membrane where they bind to and activate intracellular receptor proteins. Until activated by the steroid, the receptor is bound by a heat

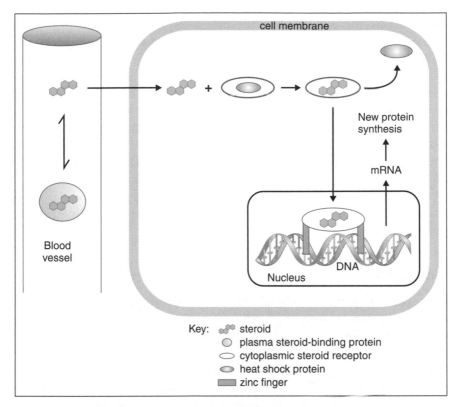

Figure 3.9 Steroid receptor mechanism of action.

shock protein, which renders the receptor unable to bind to its site of action on the genomic DNA. Binding of the steroid dissociates the receptor from the heat shock protein. This 'unmasks', on the receptor, two so-called zinc fingers, consisting of two polypeptide loops that are stabilised by Zn ions. Two activated steroid receptors dimerise and the steroid–receptor complex attaches itself to a specific hormone response element (HRE) on the DNA; this triggers transcriptional change. Therefore when steroids are used clinically their onset of action is delayed by several hours.

Biological drugs and cancer chemotherapy

The discovery of the oestrogen receptor paved the way for the synthesis of the oestrogen receptor antagonist tamoxifen by AstraZeneca, which has also proved invaluable in the ongoing elucidation of the mechanism of oestrogenic action in health and disease. Before the discovery of the oestrogen receptor and the development of tamoxifen, chemotherapy was relatively non-specific. Today, breast cancer biopsies determine whether the tumour is oestrogen receptor positive or negative. If positive, then tamoxifen is an option. Another option is the use of trastuzumab (Herceptin). This is a humanised monoclonal antibody that blocks the HER2/neu receptor (HER2 is the acronym for human epidermal growth factor receptor 2). HER receptors occur on the cell membrane and they selectively recognise mitogens and bind to them. This binding reaction triggers an intracellular response that is part of the system regulating a variety of cellular functions including cell growth and division, differentiation, adhesion and survival. Breast cancer can result from inappropriate and prolonged activation of the HER2/neu receptor, which switches on uncontrolled cell division and breast cancer.

The eventual identification of similar cell membrane receptors in prostate tissue may yield a biological approach to the treatment of, for example, prostate cancer.

Calcitonin

In humans, calcitonin is a 32-amino acid polypeptide that forms into a single α-helix. It is secreted from the C cells of the thyroid gland. When circulating calcium levels rise, calcitonin is secreted from the parafollicular cells of the thyroid gland. Its physiological role is unclear. Administered calcitonin will reduce plasma calcium by an action on osteoclasts in bone to suppress the release of calcium and phosphate, and in the gut to reduce calcium uptake. In the kidney, calcitonin inhibits calcium and phosphate reabsorption. In both tissues, the action is mediated by G-protein-coupled membrane receptors on the cell surface.

Uses

Calcitonin was used clinically to treat, for example, Paget's disease of bone, postmenopausal osteoporosis and hypercalcaemia until replaced by the bisphosphonates. It can be used as a diagnostic tumour marker for medullary thyroid adenocarcinoma, when circulating calcitonin levels are raised.

Parathyroid hormone

Parathyroid hormone (PTH) is secreted from the parathyroid glands, which are embedded in the thyroid gland. It is a linear 84-amino acid protein. PTH increases circulating Ca^{2+} levels by: (1) stimulating osteoclasts, thus promoting Ca^{2+} reabsorption from bone; (2) enhancing tubular Ca^{2+} reabsorption in the kidneys; and (3) promoting vitamin D production in the kidney – vitamin D promotes Ca^{2+} absorption in the gastrointestinal tract. PTH action is mediated by type 1 and 2 PTH receptors. Type 1 is a G-protein-coupled membrane receptor that activates both cyclic AMP and the inositol phosphate second messenger receptor systems; type 2 receptor-mediated effects may be mediated by Ca^{2+} intracellular mobilisation.

Uses of PTH

PTH is used to treat osteoporosis in postmenopausal women who are at risk of fractures, particularly in the vertebrae.

Insulin

Insulin is, at the time of writing, the only effective treatment for juvenile-onset diabetes mellitus, caused by autoimmune destruction of pancreatic islet cells. No synthetic alternatives to insulin have been found. The insulin molecule has, however, been modified using methods including recombinant DNA technology, principally in order to alter its duration of action.

Some properties of insulin

- Endocrine hormone secreted from the β cells of the pancreatic islets of Langerhans.
- Approximately 45 insulin units secreted daily from the human pancreas.
- Insulin gene occurs on the short arm of chromosome 11.
- Human insulin consists of two chains: A has 21 amino acids and B has 30 amino acids.
- The chains are linked by two disulphide bridges at A7B7 and A20B19.
- The A chain has a disulphide bridge at A6A11.
- Insulin circulates mainly as a monomer of molecular weight 6 kilodaltons (kDa).
- Insulin can form dimers of 12 kDa; when zinc is present, three dimers can form a 36-kDa hexamer.
- Insulin half-life: about 3–5 min.
- First-pass metabolism removes about 50% of insulin from the circulation.

Release and actions of insulin

Insulin is an anabolic hormone. It is released in response to rises in circulating glucose, notably postprandially (after a meal) and it reduces the blood levels of glucose by promoting:

- tissue uptake of glucose from the circulation

- in the liver, conversion of glucose to glycogen which is stored
- the production of protein and fat in the tissues.

Mechanism of action of insulin

At the metabolic level, insulin acts anabolically by activating protein phosphatases, which dephosphorylate enzymes involved in catabolic processes. Insulin thus counteracts catabolic hormones such as adrenaline and glucagon.

At the molecular level, insulin acts through autophosphorylation of its own membrane surface receptor (Figure 3.10), which triggers the rapid removal of glucose from the circulation onto the cell, where a cascade of reactions occurs, including:

- enhanced cellular uptake of glucose and amino acids
- enhanced protein and triglyceride synthesis
- inhibition of triglyceride breakdown in fat
- inhibition of hepatic gluconeogenesis.

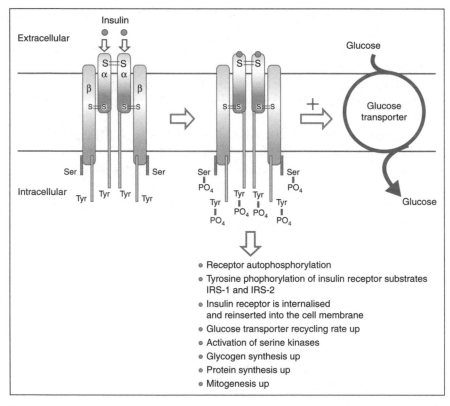

Figure 3.10   Insulin receptor action.

Intracellular signalling pathways of the insulin receptor

Activation of the insulin receptor by insulin triggers a cascade of intracellular enzymatic activations, the initial reaction being the intracellular autophosphorylation of the β subunit of the insulin receptor. The activated β subunit of the receptor in turn phosphorylates the insulin receptor substrate (IRS) proteins at multiple sites. There are two IRS molecules – IRS-1 and IRS-2 – and IRS-2 appears to be the one that mediates most of the biological effects of insulin. Phosphorylation of IRS in turn triggers the docking of several different kinases at different SH2 and SH3 sites on the IRS protein. SH2 is the acronym for the *Src* homology 2 domain of the protein, and has a strong binding affinity for phosphorylated tyrosine residues.

Examples of insulin activation

Insulin's action in promoting glucose uptake by the cell is mediated through the docking of a phosphatidylinositol-3-kinase (PI-3 kinase) at IRS-1 or 2, which triggers the translocation of glucose transporter proteins from intracellular vesicles to the cell membrane, resulting in the enhancement of glucose uptake by the cell through the glucose transporters. Insulin's anabolic action in promoting mitosis and growth is mediated in part through docking of activated IRS-1 at SH2/SH3 domains of the Grb2 protein. Grb2 is the acronym for the type 2 growth factor receptor-bound protein, and this triggers a mitogen-activated protein kinase.

Clinical use of insulin

The insulin unit

The activity contained in $^1/_{22}$ milligram of the international standard of zinc insulin crystals.

Standard strength of insulin

100 units/mL (U100).

Administration

Usually self-administered subcutaneously. Other injection devices include syringe pumps and insulin pens. Patients usually monitor their own glucose blood levels, which should ideally be kept within limits (3–7 mmol/L).

Complications of treatment with insulin

The most serious problem is hypoglycaemia through inadvertent overdose with insulin. Symptoms include tremor, dizziness, excess perspiration and syncope (fainting), which if left untreated progresses to coma, convulsions and death. If possible, glucose or sugar should be taken orally; if the patient is unconscious glucose is given slowly by infusion intravenously. Glucose should be infused slowly and with care because extravasation of glucose is an irritant to the surrounding tissues

Glucagon is also used parenterally, especially for hypotensive emergencies when the patient is comatose and cannot take glucose orally.

Insulin preparations

Previously derived from bovine or porcine sources, modern insulin preparations basically have the human amino acid sequence and can be made using recombinant DNA technology. Insulin for injection has been formulated and modified in several forms so as to provide the prescriber with options for speed of onset and duration of action. In practice, prescribers may use the different forms in combination

Short-acting insulin preparations

These are used mainly for emergencies, but can also be prescribed in combination with longer-acting formulations. They are the only forms that can be used intravenously. After subcutaneous injection, there is a delay of about 30 min before onset of action, and duration of action is variable but usually around 8 h. After intravenous injection, onset of action is rapid but of shorter duration, usually of the order of 30 min. These insulin preparations are:

- soluble insulin (also called neutral insulin), which is a solution of 100 units/mL of bovine, porcine or human insulin, pH 6.5–8
- insulin analogues:
  - insulin aspart
  - insulin glulisine
  - insulin lispro.

Intermediate-acting insulin preparations

These consist of mixtures of fast-acting and slower-acting insulin formulations. When given by subcutaneous injection, these preparations generally have an onset of action of around 1–2 h and their effective activity may last from around 15 h to 24 h.

Some currently used preparations:

- Biphasic isophane insulins: insulin complexed with the basic protein protamine, providing a range of preparations of varying onset and duration time; examples include the Humulins and Human Mixtard.

- Insulin zinc suspension (IZS): acetate-buffered mixtures of amorphous and crystalline insulin; acetate buffering prolongs action. Amorphous insulin with smaller particles of insulin has a rapid onset but shorter duration of action whereas crystalline insulin with larger particles has a slower onset but more prolonged duration. The mixture provides a smoother and more prolonged action.

Long-acting insulin preparations

- Insulin detemir: a recombinant insulin molecule with the natural insulin amino acid sequence but with a fatty acid moiety attached to the terminal β-chain amino acid. This confers fat solubility on the molecule with slower absorption from the injection site, and also higher affinity for circulating albumin, which prolongs circulation half-life.
- Insulin glargine: an acidic solution of insulin for subcutaneous injection once daily; it is injected at bedtime and deposits microcrystalline insulin which is continuously released into the bloodstream; onset of action is reached within 1 h, maximum activity within 4–6 h and activity is maintained for about 24 h.
- Protamine zinc insulin: protamine is a basic protein that forms an insoluble complex with insulin at a pH of about 8, thus forming a long-lasting, slow-release form of insulin at the site of injection. The onset of insulin's action is apparent at about 6 h after injection, and may last about 24–30 h. Protamine, being alkaline, may cause local hypersensitivity reactions.

Insulin use under certain circumstances

In certain cases, e.g. before major surgery, during serious bouts of intercurrent illness or during pregnancy, expert professional advice and supervision are required.

Clinical scenario: type 1 diabetes

Tim is a 14-year-old boy who has been well throughout childhood. His parents have been increasingly concerned over 3 weeks as he seemed to be very tired, drinking a lot of water and juice, and perhaps losing a little weight. They book an appointment with his GP, but, the night before, they become so concerned that he is rushed to accident and emergency. He is very weak and pale, complaining of central abdominal pain and breathing abnormally.

The medical staff quickly assess the situation, noting profound dehydration, very high blood sugar levels and severe metabolic acidosis, and make a diagnosis of ketoacidosis secondary to new-onset type 1 diabetes mellitus.

Tim is transferred to the high dependency unit and monitored carefully overnight. He requires rehydration with several litres of saline, and is started on an infusion of short-acting insulin. Over 2 days he makes an excellent recovery, is pacing up and down the ward, and is desperate to get home.

On the third day the consultant sits down with the family and begins the lengthy process of educating them properly about diabetes mellitus. They are dismayed that it is a life-long condition without cure, and Tim seems to be angry about the need for both regular injections and restricting his poor diet. He is prescribed an insulin regimen involving three short-acting insulin injections around mealtimes and an intermediate-acting version at bedtime; he is taught how to administer the injections himself with an autoinjecting 'pen'.

Tim is reviewed 10 days later in clinic with his blood sugar diary. His diabetes control is poor and Tim admits to finding four injections a day difficult, and often skips the lunchtime dose when mum is not around. They decide to try him on a twice-daily regimen involving a biphasic insulin preparation (i.e. a short- and intermediate-acting mix of insulins). At the next clinic appointment his blood sugar control is much better and Tim seems more accepting of the diagnosis.

Growth hormone

Growth hormone (GH) is a 191-amino acid polypeptide of molecular weight about 22 kDa, and is synthesised in the somatotroph cells of the anterior pituitary gland. The molecular structure includes four helices, which largely determine the binding specificity to the GH receptor, and two disulphide bridges. GH from other primates is active in humans but not GH from lower species.

Secretion of GH

Secretion is pulsatile, with wide variations in pulse height and frequency during a 24-hour period. Patterns and amplitudes vary within and between individuals. Surges frequently occur shortly after sleep onset, and GH release activity is often relatively high during the rapid eye movement (REM) stages of sleep.

Regulation of GH release

GH release is controlled primarily by the hypothalamus, which releases GH-releasing hormone (GHRH), and somatostatin, which inhibits GH release.

GHRH is a 44-amino acid polypeptide synthesised in the arcuate nucleus of the hypothalamus. It is released in a pulsatile pattern and is transported in the blood via the portal system to the anterior pituitary, where it binds to the GHRH receptor on anterior pituitary somatotroph cells; this stimulates GH release into the general circulation. Other stimulants to GH release include:

- amino acids, notably arginine
- androgen secretion during puberty
- exercise
- ghrelin, a polypeptide hormone secreted by the stomach, which is a potent GH-releasing agent; ghrelin is also a powerful appetite stimulant
- hypoglycaemia
- protein (dietary)
- sleep.

Somatostatin is a polypeptide released into the portal system by the periventricular nucleus of the hypothalamus; it inhibits GH release from the pituitary gonadotrophs. It also has an inhibitory action on the release of TSH. Somatostatin is produced in the gastrointestinal tract where it inhibits the release of several other gut hormones, e.g. cholecystokinin (CCK), enteroglucagon, gastrin, motilin and vasointestinal peptide (VIP).

Mechanism of action of GH

On arrival at the target cell, GH binds to a membrane receptor, which causes dimerisation of the GH receptor; this in turn causes recruitment of the intracellular tyrosine kinase JAK-2 (Janus kinase-2; this name is derived from an ancient two-faced Roman god called Janus); the activated JAK-2 kinases in turn phosphorylate and thereby activate so-called STAT proteins; the activated STAT proteins switch on nuclear transcription and cell growth and division. Other enzyme systems activated by JAK-2 include the MAPK system (MAPK – mitogen-activated protein kinase) and the PI-3 kinase, which generates a fast metabolic response by the cell.

Clinical uses of GH and somatostatin analogues

Nomenclature note: Synthetic GH prepared by recombinant DNA techniques somatropin.

In children GH is prescribed for the following:

- Children with proven deficiency of GH.
- Chronic renal insufficiency before puberty (when renal function is decreased to <50%), which leads to growth failure.
- Prader–Willi syndrome, which is a congenital problem, typically characterised by hypogonadism, hypotonia and immature sex organ development; children are somnolent and overeat (hyperphagia), leading to obesity, and have poor social and emotional development; there may be learning difficulties.
- Turner syndrome, when females are born with only one X chromosome. Such females lack ovaries. Growth is generally retarded and there may be webbing of the neck.

In adults, if there is a severe deficiency of GH associated with impaired quality of life, and if there are other anterior pituitary deficiencies the somatostatin analogues lanreotide and octreotide are used, for example, for the following:

- reducing GH secretion from anterior pituitary tumours
- treatment of thyroid tumours (lanreotide)
- preventing complications after pancreatic surgery (lanreotide)
- reduction of vomiting during palliative care (octreotide).

See the *BNF* for more details.

The incretins

The incretins, glucose-dependent insulinotropic polypeptide (GIP) and glucagon-like peptide-1 (GLP-1), are intestinal peptide hormones released by intestinal epithelium in response to glucose. The circulation transports them to the pancreas where they stimulate insulin secretion. They therefore supplement the hypoglycaemic action of insulin. The observation that oral glucose was more potent than intravenous glucose was the original impetus for this discovery. They are now of considerable interest for the treatment of type 2 diabetes mellitus, when tissues are relatively insensitive to endogenous insulin. In addition, there is evidence that GLP-1 delays gastric emptying, thus slowing the rate of glucose absorption. It also inhibits glucagon secretion. In addition, a peptide called exendin-4, with properties similar to those of GLP-1, has been identified in the saliva of the Gila monster.

The discovery of the incretins has given new impetus to the development of antidiabetic drugs.

Multiple choice questions

For each question, five options are provided and only one is correct.

1 The thyroid gland:
   a   Is situated beneath the trachea
   b   Secretes thyroglobulin
   c   Inhibits glucose absorption from the gastrointestinal tract
   d   Reduces plasma cholesterol
   e   Blocks vitamin A biosynthesis during stress

2 Thyroid hormone release from the thyroid gland:
   a   Is stimulated by hypothalamic thyroglobulin
   b   Depends on a functional positive feedback of thyroid hormone on TSH release from the anterior pituitary gland
   c   Is inhibited by TRH
   d   Is promoted by anterior pituitary TSH
   e   Is enhanced by vitamin A

3 The adrenal cortex:
   a   Is situated immediately below the kidney
   b   Secretes adrenaline (epinephrine) in response to stress
   c   Is structurally divided into upper cortical and lower medullary layers
   d   Is under the control of hypothalamic ACTH
   e   Secretes the glucocorticoids

4 Adrenaline (epinephrine):
   a   Binds to adrenoreceptors on the nuclear membrane
   b   Is used clinically as a rescue measure in cases of anaphylactic shock
   c   Will exacerbate glaucoma
   d   Is useful as an adjunct to local anaesthesia by causing local vasodilatation
   e   Slows the heart

5 The male sex hormone testosterone:
   a   Acts through cell membrane-bound receptors that activate the cyclic AMP second messenger system
   b   Has poor lipid solubility
   c   Has a very rapid onset of action
   d   Is secreted from the epididymal cells in the male
   e   Acts through intracellular receptors that promote new protein synthesis

6 Trastuzumab:
   a   Is a humanised monoclonal antibody that activates the HER2/neu receptor

b   Can be used to treat oestrogen receptor-negative breast tumours
c   Is administered orally
d   Triggers vigorous cell division
e   Exacerbates breast cancer

7 Calcitonin:

a   Is secreted from C cells of the thyroid gland
b   Increases the release of calcium into the bloodstream
c   Promotes calcium reabsorption in the kidneys
d   Is used to treat hypoglycaemia
e   Can be used as a diagnostic marker for prostate cancer

8 Insulin:

a   Is secreted from the α cells of the pancreatic islets
b   Consists of three polypeptide chains, linked by disulphide bonds
c   Is administered orally
d   Promotes glucose uptake into the tissues
e   Increases plasma glucose concentrations

9 Growth hormone:

a   Is secreted by gonadotroph cells of the anterior pituitary gland
b   Is secreted in a pulsatile fashion
c   Secretion is regulated by hypothalamic GnRH
d   Acts mainly through receptors in the mitochondria
e   Should not be prescribed for chronic renal insufficiency

Further reading

Banting FG, Best CH. The internal secretion of the pancreas. *J Lab Clin Med* 1922; 7: 465–80.

Bayliss WM, Starling EH. The mechanism of pancreatic secretion. *J Physiol (Lond)* 1902; 28: 325–53.

Hudis CA. Trastuzumab – mechanism of action and use in clinical practice. *N Engl J Med* 2007; 357: 39–51.

Murray GR. Note on the treatment of myxoedema by hypodermic injections of an extract of the thyroid gland of a sheep. *BMJ* 1891; ii: 796.

Nutton E. The rise of medicine. In: Porter R (ed.), *The Cambridge History of Medicine*. Cambridge: Cambridge University Press, 2006, 46–70.

Popa G, Fielding U. A portal system from the pituitary to the hypothalamic region. *J Anat* 1930; 65(Pt1): 88–91.

Widernman RD, Kieffer IJ. Mining incretin hormone pathways for novel therapies. *Trends Endocrinol Metab* 2009; 20: 280–6.

4

The nature of inflammation and mediators of inflammation

Objectives:

- Be able to give a definition of inflammation and the main terms, e.g. allergen, antibody.
- Know the classification of the four main types of hypersensitivity, examples and their respective causes (or theories of causes) and symptoms.
- Be able to provide examples of tissue and organ hypersensitivity responses in terms of symptoms.
- Know the symptoms of asthma.
- Have a basic knowledge of aetiology of haemolytic disease of the newborn.
- Know the given mechanisms and chemical mediators of the inflammatory response.
- Classify the protein cytokines and growth factors.
- Have good grounding in the nature, occurrence, release, mechanism of action and effects of TNF-α.
- Know the clinical implications of TNF-α.
- Know the nature and clinical significance of the chemokines and their receptors.
- Be able to give examples of the interleukins, namely their occurrence, target cells and actions, and therapeutic relevance.
- Know the nature, classification and actions of some of the clinical uses of the interferons.

Inflammation may be defined as a response of the body to injury. The response may be acute or chronic. Physical trauma, chemical agents or infection may initiate an inflammatory response. The initial response is usually characterised by redness at the site of inflammation and warmth, pain and swelling.

Another sign might be the exudation of fluids. Inflammation may result in mild-to-severe loss of certain bodily functions, e.g. loss of mobility in severe cases of rheumatoid arthritis.

Traditionally, the inflammatory response was classified into two components, namely the cellular and exudative components. The exudative component describes the composition and movement of fluids from blood vessels into the tissues and the cellular component describes the movement and different functions of the leukocytes.

Inflammation was thought, among other things, to be simply the symptom of damage to the tissues, or of infection, but it is now known to be the tangible signs of the body's complex protective response to the noxious stimulus. Inflammation is a coordinated mobilisation of the body's healing mechanisms, and without it the survival of the organism could be seriously compromised. Once the inflammatory process has done its work there may be no sign of the original trauma or of the inflammatory response; a more severe trauma could result in the formation of scar tissue.

Normally, the body does not allow the inflammatory response to outlive its useful work, but in some cases the it seems to uncouple from the normal control system's healing mechanism and 'run wild'. Manifestations of this uncoupling include relatively mild chronic conditions such as hay fever, and more serious chronic inflammatory conditions such as systemic lupus erythematosus (SLE), rheumatoid arthritis (RA) and scleroderma. It is not yet precisely known what causes the immune system to identify as foreign and attack the tissues of the same organism, and this is a question the answer to which may point the way to the most appropriate and successful treatment of autoimmune diseases

Hypersensitivity

The term 'hypersensitivity' is widely used to describe an inappropriate or excessively large inflammatory response of the organism to a noxious or damaging stimulus. The stimulus may be chemical, e.g. dietary albumin in egg, pollen, drugs or chemicals in, for example, insect bites and stings or in animal fur. It may be mechanical, through tissue injury. It is necessary here to consider the mechanisms of hypersensitivity in view of the immunogenic potential of many of the biological drugs used. Four types of hypersensitivity have traditionally been defined (although this is a mildly controversial classification) in terms of the lag time to initiation of onset of the reaction:

1 Type I: anaphylactic or immediate hypersensitivity
2 Type II: cytotoxic hypersensitivity
3 Type III: immune complex hypersensitivity
4 Type IV: delayed or cell-mediated hypersensitivity (not recognised by some authorities).

Type I hypersensitivity

Type I is the relatively rapid response to an allergen, e.g. insect bite, food, e.g. egg albumin or a drug, e.g. penicillin, and symptoms include urticaria (itchy skin rash) and local redness [vasodilatation] and swelling [oedema]), caused by local histamine release from mast cells. The tissue response results from the reaction between a pre-existing IgE antibody and the allergen, and the consequent acute inflammatory events notably include:

- smooth muscle contraction
- enhanced vascular permeability
- extravasation of cells and plasma fluid into the tissues
- granulocyte chemotaxis
- activation of mast cells.

Tissue and organ responses include some or all of these symptoms:

- skin: eczema, urticaria
- gut: gastroenteritis
- eyes: conjunctival symptoms
- bronchopulmonary tract: symptoms of asthma.

The mechanism, basically, involves the action of the allergen, also called the antigen (e.g. egg albumin), which stimulates the production of IgE antibodies that are directed specifically against that antigen. The IgE antibody thus produced has a high affinity for its receptors on basophils and mast cells, and the net result of the binding reaction is the release of histamine and other mediators into the surrounding tissues or the systemic circulation. Histamine in the general circulation can cause a profound and potentially fatal fall in blood pressure and very severe bronchoconstriction. Treatment here may include cardiopulmonary resuscitation and administration of adrenaline in the case of anaphylactic shock.

The lag time to initiation of the response is around 2.5–35 min.

Type II hypersensitivity

This is sometimes referred to as cytotoxic hypersensitivity. In type II hypersensitivity, the antibodies involved are IgG and IgM. Three main type II reactions are defined:

1 Blood transfusion reactions
2 Drug-induced hypersensitivity
3 Haemolytic disease of the newborn.

Blood transfusion reactions

These reactions occur because of variability of blood groups between individuals with particular reference to the glycosylation of certain red blood cell glycoproteins, namely the ABO group. The four blood groups are A, B, O and AB. If, for example, a type A individual with circulating anti-B antibodies is injected with type B blood, these blood cells will agglutinate and burst the foreign cells.

Drug-induced hypersensitivity

This may be caused by drugs of relatively small molecular weight, e.g. aspirin, which alone are too small to stimulate antibody production, but can bind covalently to platelets or red blood cells, thereby creating an antigen. In this case aspirin is referred to as a hapten. The molecule thus formed stimulates an immune response, which can result in, for example, anaemia, opsonisation or thrombocytopenia, depending on the drug involved.

Haemolytic disease of the newborn

Red blood cells possess on their surface an antigen called the rhesus (Rh) antigen. Most people are Rh positive (Rh+), but a smaller percentage of the population lack the antigen and are termed Rh negative (Rh−). A potential danger exists, because red blood cells can cross the placenta between the mother and the fetus.

   During childbirth, some of the baby's red cells do cross the placenta and enter the mother's circulation. If a Rh− mother produces an Rh+ baby, then blood cells passing from the baby to the mother will cause the mother's immune system to produce IgG antibodies to the Rh antigen. If the mother then subsequently falls pregnant with another Rh+ fetus, the mother's anti-Rh IgG, which passes easily across the placenta, will enter the baby's bloodstream and recognise and bind to Rh on the baby's blood cells. This can cause opsonisation, whereby the cell becomes a candidate for phagocytosis and destruction in the spleen and liver, with the generation of toxic levels of bilirubin. If an Rh− mother is identified in time, she can be treated with anti-D immunoglobulin, which prevents her immune system from recognising Rh.

   The lag time to onset of initiation of the reaction is around 4–9 h.

Type III hypersensitivity (immune complex hypersensitivity)

This form of hypersensitivity is mediated through the actions of soluble immune complexes, principally IgG, and also complement, notably C3a, C4a, C5a. The disease may affect individual organs, e.g. the kidneys, lung or skin, or affect the body generally. The causative factor may be exogenous, e.g. infections by viruses, bacteria or parasites, or endogenous (autoimmune) diseases. Examples of diseases produced include the Arthus reaction, aspergillosis, RA, SLE and polyarteritis. The antibodies involved in the hypersensitivity are IgG or IgM antibodies.

Systemic immune complex disease, also called serum disease, is an example of type III hypersensitivity, and may occur when an animal-derived antiserum, e.g. anti-tetanus or diphtheria, is given to a human. The foreign proteins in the serum can generate a powerful antibody response in the human recipient, and the second dose of antiserum can precipitate an inflammatory response when the antibodies thus formed recognise proteins in a subsequent dose of vaccine and bind to them. The complexes bind to blood vessel walls, including in the skin, joints and internal organs, e.g. the kidneys. And they fix complement, largely due to activation of tumour necrosis factor (TNF)-α-producing T cells.

The lag time to initiation of onset of the reaction is around 1.5–10 h.

Type IV hypersensitivity

(Not all authorities accept the validity of the use of a fourth class of hypersensitivity.)

This is also termed, in some texts, 'delayed-type hypersensitivity' or 'cell-mediated hypersensitivity'.

Mechanisms and chemical mediators of the inflammatory response

It is worth considering the mechanisms and chemical mediators of the inflammatory response, because this knowledge has made possible the development and use of many, if not most, of the currently available biological drugs, and several more are undoubtedly in the pipeline.

Tissue damage triggers activation of cells in the tissue, notably resident macrophage cells; the nature of the cells depends on the tissue. Kuppfer's cells, for example, are liver macrophages, and dendritic cells occur mainly in tissues in close proximity to the external environment, e.g. skin and mucosal tissue. Mastocytes, or mast cells, are present in several different tissues. When activated, these cells release inflammatory mediator chemicals, including histamine, cytokines, interleukins, notably IL-2 and IL-6, as well as TNF-α. These mediators cause vasodilatation and increase vascular permeability, which allows the escape of fluids and white cells from the blood into the damaged tissue. Some are also chemotactic, in that they attract monocytes and neutrophils to the site of inflammation. These events produce the symptoms of redness and oedema.

Protein cytokines

Cytokines are proteins or peptides that are released by cells in response to antigenic activation of the cell. They play a critical role in the functions of the adaptive and innate members of the immune system. Once released, cytokines bind to specific receptors on the surface of cells of the immune system. Some members can be classed in more than one category.

Protein cytokines, for the current purposes, may be classified as:

- primary effector cytokines, e.g. TNF-α and IL-1: these, alone, can induce serious inflammatory reactions
- chemokines, e.g. chemokine receptor 1 (CCR1)
- interleukins, e.g. IL-2
- growth factors, e.g. epidermal growth factor (EGF)
- interferons, e.g. interferon-α.

The cytokines are targets for biological anti-inflammatory drugs. As soon as the initial stimulus to the acute phase of inflammation is removed the acute phase will rapidly cease, mainly due to the relatively short half-lives of the chemical mediators of inflammation. In chronic inflammatory conditions, there is rampant and uncontrolled activity of these factors, notably of TNF-α, which is a prominent target for the biological anti-inflammatory drugs (see below).

Tumour necrosis factor-α

TNF-α belongs to a superfamily of molecules with the primary role of regulation of cell survival. At least 19 members of the TNF family are known at the time of writing, and at least 29 receptors have been identified for this superfamily. TNF-α and other members of this superfamily are normally protective by, among other actions, blocking tumorigenesis, causing apoptosis and blocking proliferation of viruses; they are used clinically to enhance immune function.

> The TNF superfamily is a huge and rapidly growing topic of considerable academic and clinical importance.

TNF-α can also destroy tissues because it is, along with other immunostimulants such as IL-2, inappropriately activated in autoimmune diseases, e.g. Crohn's disease and RA.

Occurrence, production and release of TNF-α

TNF-α is produced principally by macrophages, but also by many other tissues including lymphocytes, adipose tissue, cardiac myocytes, endothelial cells, fibroblasts and cells of the nervous system. The stimuli for TNF-α release from these cells include IL-1 and lipopolysaccharides of bacterial origin.

TNF-α structure and biosynthesis

TNF-α is biosynthesised as a type II transmembrane protein consisting of 212 amino acids arranged in the form of homotrimers. A homotrimer here is a polypeptide composed of three exactly identical polypeptide units. TNF-α is a pleotropic molecule, which means that it can exert multiple effects and can exist in more than one form. (*Nomenclature note*: a type I transmembrane protein is usually positioned such that its amino-terminal end is external to the membrane; type II transmembrane protein has its carboxy-terminal end external to the cell membrane.)

TNF-α is released from the membrane through a proteolytic cleavage reaction catalysed by a metalloprotease enzyme called TNF-α-converting enzyme (TACE).

Mechanism of action of TNF-α

Two receptors specific for TNF-α have been identified at the time of writing, namely TNF-α R1 and TNF-α R2. Type R1 is expressed by many tissues and both the membrane-bound form and the soluble form of TNF-α can activate R1. R2, on the other hand, occurs selectively in cells of the immune system, and is activated only by membrane-bound TNF-α.

Actions of TNF-α

TNF-α acts on many tissues, including the brain, liver, pancreas and macrophages, generally in concert with IL-1 and IL-6:

- Macrophages: TNF-α acts on macrophages to promote phagocytosis and the production of inflammatory mediators, e.g. prostaglandins $F_{2\alpha}$ and E_2.
- Brain: TNF-α together with IL-6 causes pyrexia (fever), suppresses appetite and stimulates the release of corticotrophin-releasing hormone (CRH) from hypothalamic neurons, resulting in increased ACTH and cortisol release.
- Liver: TNF-α activates many different intracellular hepatic pathways. It regulates cellular proliferation, apoptosis (programmed cell death) and hepatic inflammation. Not only is it potentially destructive in liver, but it also promotes liver regeneration.
- Chemotaxis: TNF-α is a powerful chemoattractant for neutrophils.
- Insulin resistance: TNF-α can cause insulin resistance in several tissues.

Clinical implications of TNF-α

TNF-α is implicated in the aetiology of several inflammatory disorders, including ankylosing spondylitis, Crohn's disease, psoriasis, refractory asthma and RA. This knowledge has made possible the development of treatments designed specifically to block the actions of TNF-α, e.g. adalimumab, etanercept and infliximab (see Chapters 5 and 6).

Some other members of the TNF-α superfamily-receptor pairs include:

- CD70L–CD27: CD70L is expressed by several cells including antigen-presenting cells (APCs), CD4+, CD8+, mast cells, natural killer (NK) cells and smooth muscle cells, and expression is induced by, for example, B-cell receptors, CD40 and interferon-γ.
- 4-IBB ligand–4-IBB receptor: 4-BB ligand is expressed by cells including CD4+, CD8+ cells, B cells and macrophages, and expression is triggered by, for example, CD40, mast cells and NK cells.
- OX40L–OX40R: OX40 ligand is expressed by cells including APCs, B cells, mast cells and NK cells, and expression is triggered by, for example, TLR2 (toll-like cell receptor 2) and DR3 (death receptor 3).

The term 'cluster of differentiation' is used to describe a large number of cell surface proteins on cells of the immune system, notably of leukocytes. The function of these proteins is usually as a type of receptor for a signalling ligand, or as a mediator of adhesion reactions, e.g. CD4 is a co-receptor on the cell surface, which enhances the ability of the T-cell receptor (TCR) to activate the T cell when it encounters an APC.

Chemokines

Chemokines are a group of chemoattractant peptides and proteins, most of which can attract white cells. They activate and recruit leukocytes into tissues. They may also be able to attract carcinogenic cells to distant sites and may therefore be important in metastatic cancers They are critically important in the aetiology of many types of acute and chronic inflammation, and in some infectious diseases. The first chemokine described was interleukin-8 (IL-8 – see below).

At least four major subfamilies of chemokines have been identified, namely CC, CXC (IL-8), –C– and CX_3C–. This refers to the arrangement of the initial two cysteine residues: CXC signifies that the two C residues are separated by another amino acid whereas CC signifies that there is no intervening amino acid. CX_3C signifies that three amino acids separate two cysteine residues. CC and –CXC– also differ in the nature of the cells that they attract. CC chemokines usually attract basophils, eosinophils, lymphocytes and monocytes, whereas –CXC– usually attracts neutrophils. Lymphotactin, a member of the –C– group, attracts mainly lymphocytes. Fractalkine, a member of the CX_3C family, attracts mainly NK cells. In addition, the –CXC– family has been further subdivided into ELR–CXC– and non-ELR–CXC–. The ELR motif is the N-terminal amino acid sequence Glu–Leu–Arg, which enables these chemokines to attract and activate neutrophils.

Note: these classifications do not cleanly delineate the various groups of protein cytokines. The interleukin IL-8, for example, is also a member of the chemokine –CXC– family.

Clinical significance of the chemokines

The chemokines are vitally important in several biosystems and play an important role in inflammation. They are important in, for example:

- angiogenesis and angiostasis
- cell recruitment
- development of the lymphoid organs and tissues
- inflammation
- lymphoid trafficking
- metastasis
- T-helper 1 (Th1)/Th2 development
- wound healing.

Chemokine receptors

Chemokine receptors are, typically, transmembrane receptors composed of seven transmembrane units, which are coupled to membrane G-proteins. Based on the type of chemokine that they bind, they are classified, logically, as CXCR1–5, CCR1–9, XCR1 and CX_3CR1.

Given the wide range of chemokine actions, their receptors are now actively sought, discovered and characterised, as well as the nature of their reactions with their ligands. This work has profound clinical implications in the search of drugs for the treatment of, for example, ovarian dysfunction, cancer metastasis and inflammation. This work is dealt with in more detail in relevant chapters, but a small range of examples of human chemokine receptors and their ligands is given in Table 4.1.

RANTES

This is a cytokine that attracts lymphocytes and memory T lymphocytes. It is also known as CCL5 and binds to a receptor called CCR5, which is a

Table 4.1 Human chemokine receptors and ligands		
Receptor	**Ligand**	**Function (example)**
CXCR1	CXC (IL-8)	Neutrophil activation
CCR1	RANTES	Chemotactic for basophils, eosinophils and T cells; recruits leukocytes to inflammation sites
CX3CR1	Fractalkine (CX3C)	Leukocyte migration and adhesion

IL, interleukin.

co-receptor of HIV. RANTES is an acronym for regulated on activation, normal T expressed and secreted.

The interleukins

The interleukins are cytokines, a large group of polypeptides, and derive their name from the fact that they were first discovered in leukocytes, but are now known to be synthesised by many different tissues, including endothelial cells, macrophages and CD4+ T lymphocytes. Many of their immunological functions have been identified (Table 4.2), and a rapidly growing number of biological drugs designed to target them and mediators involved in their synthesis and action are now in use or being developed.

The present system of mediator classification is probably under review because several mediators may be co-classified as lymphokines, cytokines and chemokines.

The process of formation of the interleukins is complex and dependent on the activation of naïve T cells and the actions of other interleukins.

For purposes of presentation the interleukins are presented separately in Table 4.2, although their actions are normally integrated, sometimes dependent on each other and in health are balanced to achieve protection form external influences, e.g. viruses, bacteria and parasitic attack.

The interferons

The interferons (IFNs) are a group of biological compounds with antiviral activity, which are used in medicine as antiviral treatments. They have other uses, e.g. in the treatment of inflammation. They are now routinely used to treat, for example, chronic hepatitis B and C (IFN-α) and relapsing–remitting multiple sclerosis (IFN-β) – see later chapters.

The nature and classification of interferons

Interferons are antiviral cytokines. They are important for the body's protective strategies against invading viruses. They were first reported in the 1950s during studies of responses in chick cells to experimental viral infection, and they have provided insights into the mechanisms whereby cells respond to viral attack and, most importantly, how viruses adapt to and overcome the body's defences. They are also important modulators of immune responses and have effects on cell differentiation, growth and immune responses.

Interferons are a relatively small cytokine family, and three main groups have been defined: type 1, 2 and 3 (currently a controversial group).

Table 4.2 Examples of interleukins (IL) and IL families

IL	Cellular/organ occurrence	Target cells and actions	Therapeutic relevance (includes antibodies)
IL-1 superfamily: 11 members identified: best understood: IL-1α, IL-1β, IL-1RA (receptor antagonist), IL-18	Adipose tissue B cells, dendritic cells Macrophages Monocytes	B cells: maturation and proliferation Macrophages: inflammatory NK (natural killer) cells: activated T-helper (Th) cells: co-stimulated	IL-1 antibody for: diabetes, gout, rheumatoid arthritis (RA): recombinant IL-1 receptor anakinra (Kineret)
IL-2	Th1 cells	Growth and activation of B-cell and T-cell responses Macrophages NK cells Oligodendrocytes	Aldesleukin (Proleukin) For metastatic renal cell carcinoma
IL-3	Activated Th cells Endothelial tissue Eosinophils Mast cells NK cells	Haematopoietic stem cells: Differentiation and proliferation of progenitor cells to, for example, erythrocytes Mast cells: histamine release	Under investigation
IL-4	Macrophages, mast cells, memory CD4+ cells, naïve, newly activated CD4+ cells, Th2 cells	B cell activated by interaction with an activated antigen	Note in IgG, IgE synthesis
IL-5	Eosinophils, mast cells, Th2 cells	B cells; cellular differentiation, production of IgA	Possible use of anti-IL-5 antiserum in asthma and eosinophilia
IL-6	Adipose tissue, astrocytes, B cells Endothelial cells Macrophages Th2 cells (subset of helper-inducer T lymphocytes)	B cells > plasma cells Antibody secretion from plasma cells Acute phase inflammatory reactions; possible role in aetiology of type 2 diabetes In RA note in chronic inflammation and joint damage	Possible use to limit ventilator-induced injury to lung alveolar barrier system Impending introduction in the UK of tocilizumab, a humanised anti-IL-6 receptor antibody for RA

(continued overleaf)

Table 4.2 *Continued*

IL	Cellular/organ occurrence	Target cells and actions	Therapeutic relevance (Includes antibodies)
IL-7	Bone marrow, thymus	Pre-/pro-B and T cells; NK cells; lymphoid progenitor cell protection	Possible use in idiopathic CD4 lymphocytopenia
IL-8 (a chemokine; see text)	Endothelial, epithelial cells; lymphocytes, macrophages	Basophils, lymphocytes, neutrophils; chemotaxis of neutrophils	Possible diagnostic tool: raised IL-8 in pregnancy associated with schizophrenia in offspring
IL-9	CD4+ helper cells, mast cells, Th2 cells	B cells, T cells; stimulation of mast cells; inhibition of apoptosis; potentiation of IgE < IgG, IgM; proinflammatory in asthma through eosinophil potentiation	Possible use of IL-9 antibodies to inhibit eosinophil action in asthma
IL-10 family (includes IL-10, -19, -20, -22, -24, -26, -28α, -28β, -29)	B cells, CD8+ T cells, Th2 cells, macrophages, monocytes	B cells: activation; Macrophages: cytokine synthesis; Th2 cells	Possible anti-tumour action
IL-11	Bone marrow stromal cells	Uterine blastocyst implantation	Possible IL-11 receptor antagonists for contraception
IL-12 family: IL-12, -23, -27	B cells, dendritic cells, macrophages, T cells, monocytes	Proinflammatory cytokines; note IL-12 is stimulator of interferon (IFN)-γ synthesis; IL-27 induces Th1 cells from naïve T cells; IL-23 is for induction of Th17 cells; all activate the JAK-STAT signalling pathways; mice deficient in IL-12 are more likely to get autoimmune inflammatory diseases	Potential targets for anti-inflammatory drugs; IL-12 antibody possible treatment for multiple sclerosis
IL-13	Mast cells, NK cells, activated Th2 cells	B cells, macrophages, Th2 cells; note role in asthma by, for example, promoting IgE synthesis by B cells, and activation of inflammatory cells through chemotaxis and induction of eosinophilia, and promotion of subepithelial fibrosis	Possible modulator of immune responses (see also IL-23)
IL-14 Two forms: α and β	B-cell lymphomas, follicular dendritic cells, T cells	Promotion of B-cell antibody production, survival, memory and growth; possibly involved in transplant rejection	IL-14 and/or receptors possible targets to treat autoimmune disorders

IL-15	Muscle, mainly by myocytes; mRNA expressed by many different tissues, including macrophages during viral infection, mononuclear phagocytes	Supports NK T-lymphocyte proliferation; inhibits muscle cell degradation; decreases fat deposition (in rodents in vivo); possibly involved in regulating adipose tissue metabolism and muscle:fat ratio; antiapoptotic; may be proinflammatory in rheumatoid arthritis and inflammatory bowel disease; may preserve muscle mass	Potential uses: e.g. potential target for anti-inflammatory treatments and in regulation of adipose tissue; potential for promotion and preservation of muscle mass
IL-16 (also called lymphocyte chemoattractant factor); biosynthesis is enhanced in inflammation and by factors including IL-1β and IL-17 (see below)	Several cell types, including CD8+ T cells, eosinophils, epithelial cells, lymphocytes and in joints by CD68− fibroblast-like cells of the synovial lining	Chemoattractant for and activator of cells, which express CD4+, a cell surface factor, e.g. dendritic cells, eosinophils and monocytes; note in inflammatory conditions, e.g. RA; inhibitor of viral replication; possible involvement in aetiology of systemic lupus erythematosus (SLE); enhances airway inflammation in bronchial asthma	Blocking IL-16 action may be beneficial in RA, SLE and bronchial asthma
IL-17 family: IL-17A to IL-17F, which has isoforms IL-17F 1 and 2	Th17 cells – CD4+ T cells	Very highly proinflammatory; important in the allergic response; involved in host defences against invading pathogens; note in aetiology of, for example, RA for antigen-specific antibody production and antigen-specific T-cell responses; may be noted in initiation of RA and in responsiveness of collagen-specific B and T cells to other inflammatory mediators, e.g. cytokines; IL-17 alone or with toll-like receptor 2 (TLR-2[a]) may exacerbate and accelerate progression of RA by increasing production of IL-16	Potential serum markers in allergic responses
IL-18: member of IL-1 superfamily	Macrophages; adrenal cells during stress; many tissues may produce these under stress	Target receptors include IL-18R1; CDw218a; promotes NK cell activity, induces IFN-γ production; highly orally inflammatory in autoimmune diseases	Receptors are possible targets for anti-inflammatory drugs
IL-19: member of IL-10 family (see above)	B cells and resting monocytes	Binds to same receptor as IL-20 and IL-24 (IL-20R1/R2), upregulated in monocytes by, for example, lipopolysaccharides; stimulates synthesis of IL-10 production in monocytes; implicated in allergic reactions and psoriasis, a Th1-type skin disease; involved in skin development	Potential tool for treatment of psoriasis
IL-20: member of IL-10 family	Expressed mainly by keratinocytes and monocytes	Binds to same receptors as IL-19; high concentrations in psoriasis and RA synovial fluid; implicated in skin development, haematopoiesis, angiogenesis and atherosclerosis	Anti-IL-20 antibody currently undergoing clinical trials for RA

(continued overleaf)

Table 4.2 Continued

IL	Cellular/organ occurrence	Target cells and actions	Therapeutic relevance (includes antibodies)
IL-21: pleotropic cytokine (can exist in more than one form)	Derived from activated CD4 T cells	Receptor: IL-21R; implicated in hypersensitivity reactions, especially allergic dermatitis; also note components of CD4+ T cell help in, for example, controlling chronic viral infection	Possible future direction for allergic dermatitis treatment; perhaps contributes to antiviral developments
IL-22: member of IL-10 family	Expressed by activated T cells and activated NK cells; CD4+ Th cells	T-cell possession of IL-22 suggests a role of IL-22 in T-cell-mediated diseases, e.g. Crohn's disease, psoriasis, interstitial lung diseases and RA; the IL-22 receptor complex is a heterodimer complex of IL-22R1–IL-10R2, found mainly in tissues of digestive and respiratory systems, kidney and skin	Possible strategies for treatment of T-cell-mediated diseases, e.g. Crohn's disease, psoriasis, interstitial lung diseases and RA
IL-3: heterodimer; some structural similarities with IL-12 (both share the P40 subunit)	Expressed by macrophages and activated dendritic cells	Promotes inflammation through promotion of pathogenic memory CD4+ T cells, which release TNF-α, IL-6 and IL-17; both IL-12 and IL-23 activate STAT4, a transcription activator, and stimulate production of IFN-γ; IL-23 receptor consists of a an IL-23-specific subunit IL-23R and the bi-subunit of the IL-12 receptor	May be useful tools for development of treatments for inflammatory bowel disease and multiple sclerosis
IL-24: member of IL-10 family	Originally found in healthy but not cancerous melanocytes and its gene found to have structural similarities with the gene for IL-10; expressed by monocytes and Th2 lymphocytes	The IL-24 receptor consists of a receptor that is a complex of IL-20R1 and IL-20R2 chains; activation causes activation of STAT3; note in, among others, development and apoptosis of tumour cells, without apparently affecting non-tumour tissue	Interesting possibilities for tumour-shrinking drug development
IL-25: member of IL-17 family (IL-17E; receptor: IL-17-RB); single transmembrane protein with homology to IL-17	Secreted by mast cells, Th2 cells	IL-25 induces airway hyperreactivity and is implicated in asthma possibly through induction of Th2 responses via invariant NK T cells, which express the IL-25 receptor (IL-17RB) IL-12 production in gut; IL-12 is implicated in ulcerative colitis	IL-25 may be a basis for treatment in inflammatory conditions of the gut, and blocking its actions in the lung may be a treatment for inflammatory lung conditions

IL-26: originally called AK155, IL-26 is a member of the IL-10 family; similar amino acid sequence to IL-10	Secreted mainly by memory T cells and monocytes; IL-6R is a complex formed of IL-10R2 and IL-20R1	Induces rapid phosphorylation of transcription factors STAT1 and STAT3, resulting in increased IL-8 and IL-10 secretion; also acts on epithelial cells to increase expression of the CD4 molecule; in gut epithelial cells, appears to be proinflammatory in, for example, Crohn's disease	Possible use of IL-26 monoclonal antibody in inflammatory gastrointestinal tract disorders
IL-27: see IL-12			
IL-28A, IL-28B, IL-29 family; some structural similarities with IL-10 family and type 1 interferons	Sources: IL-29: monocytes; dendritic cells challenged by bacteria secrete IL-28 and IL-29. Viral attack also stimulates IL-28 and IL-29 production	Receptors for IL-28 and IL-29: a heterodimeric cytokine receptor composed of IL-10R and an orphan class II receptor chain called IL-28R. Antiviral interferon receptors for IFN 1, 2 and 3 identified, possibly as complexes of orphan class II receptor IL-28R and receptor IL-10Rb	This class of interleukins may provide basis for immunity to infection by viruses
IL-30: forms part of IL-27, so also called IL27-p28; structurally resembles IL-6			
IL-31: structurally related to IL-6 family	Synthesised by Th2 cells	Receptor is a complex of oncostatin M receptor subunits and IL-31RA; may be involved in skin inflammation; over-expressed in pruritic atopic skin lesions	Possible target for treatment of skin disorders such as eczema
IL-32: structurally unrelated to other cytokine families; originally induced in tissues by IL-18 and called NK4	IL-32 mRNA is expressed in, for example, B cells, monocytes, activated peripheral T cells and lymphoid tissues	An inflammatory cytokine; induces TNF-α, IL-1β and IL-6 expression in vitro and in vivo; has at least six isoforms; low levels expressed in healthy tissues, but high expression in many different inflamed tissues in inflammation, e.g. Crohn's disease, chronic obstructive pulmonary disease and RA	Potentially powerful tool in development of biological anti-inflammatory treatments

(continued overleaf)

Table 4.2 *Continued*

IL	Cellular/organ occurrence	Target cells and actions	Therapeutic relevance (Includes antibodies)
IL-33: member of IL-1 superfamily; originally described in high endothelial venules (HEVs) and called NF-κB (HEVs facilitate entry of lymphocytes into lymphoid tissue from the circulation)	Receptors: IL-R1 and IL-1 RAP[b]	IL-33 receptor is an orphan receptor of the IL-1 family, namely IL-1 receptor T2, which activates intracellular MAP kinases and NF-κB *in vivo*; IL-33 induces the expression of the IL-4, -5 and -13; known to inflame mucosal tissue	Potentially important for development of treatments that block its actions, especially in mucosal organs
IL-34: relatively newly discovered interleukin and identification of its receptor; structurally unrelated to other cytokines	Receptor identified as colony-stimulating-1 receptor (CSF-1R)	Expressed in several tissues, including brain, heart, kidney, liver, ovary, spleen, and testis. Actions: Selectively increases production of and activates and increases viability of primary monocytes	IL-34 could form basis for enhancement of monocytes differentiation, proliferation and survival
IL-35: relatively new cytokine related to the IL-12 family; produced by fusion of p35 subunit of IL-12A and IL-27b; produced by regulatory T cells, a subset of CD4+ T cells that inhibit development of autoimmunity	IL-35 receptors: little is known at time of writing	Actions: IL-35 is anti-inflammatory; suppresses immune responses through proliferation of T$_{reg}$ cells, a subpopulation of CD4+ T cells that prevent the development of autoimmunity, and suppression of Th17 cells, which release Th17 that is highly implicated in autoimmune disease	Potential tool for use in autoimmune diseases

[a] Toll-like receptor 2 (TLR-2) is a membrane-spanning receptor that recognises bacteria.
[b] RAP, receptor accessory protein.
RA, rheumatoid arthritis.

Type 1 interferons

Type 1 interferons are principally antiviral in function, mainly by blocking viral replication. There are, in humans, three members of this group, namely IFN-α, IFN-β and IFN-ω. Several subtypes of IFN-α have been described, all of which bind to a cell surface receptor complex, called the IFN-α receptor (IFNAR). The receptor is made up of one chain consisting of two subunits, namely IFNAR1 and IFNAR2. An important intracellular pathway activated by this receptor (and by the other interferon types) is the JAK-STAT signalling pathway. Other intracellular pathways activated by the interferons include the phosphatidylinositol 3-kinase and mitogen-activated protein kinase p38 cascades.

Production

IFN-α and IFN-β are produced by several different cells, including B cells, fibroblasts, NK cells, T cells and by plasmacytoid dendritic cell precursors (pDCs), which are a specialised form of circulating monocytes. The pDCs express toll-like receptors TLR-7 and TLR-9. Toll-like receptors constitute a vital part of the mechanisms involved in the recognition of factors produced by microorganisms and the activation of host defence mechanisms.

Type 2 interferon

Only one type 2 interferon is currently described, namely IFN-γ. IFN-γ binds to the IFN-γ receptor (IFNGR). This is a cell surface receptor consisting of two subunits, namely IFNGR1 and IFNGR2. This interferon is of great importance for the proper functioning of both adaptive and innate immunity. Abnormalities of IFN-γ activity are associated with autoimmune diseases, including inflammatory diseases. This interferon is therefore of interest in the search for treatments for, for example, RA and Crohn's disease.

Type 3 interferons

A controversial class – not universally accepted.

Some important actions of interferons

- Antiviral
- Anti-oncogenic
- Activation of macrophage and NK-cell activity
- Enhance presentation of exogenous (foreign) peptide sequences to T cells
- Anti-inflammatory – IFN-β
- Proinflammatory – IFN-γ

IFN-α has been reported, among other things, to:

- be a powerful antiviral agent
- modulate immune responses to both self and foreign antigens
- be released from APC cells as an early response to antigen presentation to T (helper) cells
- provide a crucial signal that generates T-helper precursor differentiation in favour of a Th1 immune response
- render Th1 cells responsive to IL-12, which increases production of IFN-γ
- modulate antibody production
- be crucial in the amplification of the CD8+ T-cell response.

IFN-β has been reported to:

- activate NK cells
- downregulate major histocompatibility complex (MHC) II expression in tumour cells and also on virus-infected cells
- upregulate transforming growth factor (TGF)-β receptor 2 (TGF-β_2) and TGF-β_1
- inhibit T-cell proliferation
- enhance T-cell cytotoxicity
- downregulate the activity of basic fibroblast growth factor at both transcriptional and translational levels, thus inhibiting angiogenesis, which is important for tumour growth.

Clinical use of interferons

Interferons have been used for several years with variable success.

- IFN-α is licensed in the UK:
  - as an adjunct to surgery for malignant melanoma
  - to treat chronic hepatitis B and C
  - to treat chronic myelogenous leukaemia
  - to treat follicular lymphoma
  - to treat hairy cell leukaemia
  - for maintenance of remission in multiple myeloma
  - to treat metastases of carcinoid tumours of the liver and lymph.
- IFN-β is licensed in the UK for treatment of relapsing–remitting multiple sclerosis and has been claimed to slow the rate of progression and relapse of the disease, and the development of disability. This may be due to downregulation by IFN-β of TNF-α and IL-1β, both of which are proinflammatory.

The *BNF* recommends caution with IFN-β in patients with a history of cardiac disease and severe myelodepression, and is absolutely contraindicated during pregnancy and breast-feeding and in patients with severe depression or expressed suicidal intention. The National Institute for Health and Clinical Excellence (NICE) does not, in principle, recommend the use of IFN-β in patients with depression.

Multiple choice questions

For each question, a maximum of five options is provided and only one is correct.

1 The inflammatory response:
   a   Is the body's reaction to trauma
   b   Involves the movement of fluids from the inflamed area to the circulation
   c   Always seriously threatens survival through physically traumatised tissue
   d   Does not involve chemical mediators
   e   Is an ill-tempered reaction to pain

2 Hypersensitivity:
   a   Always includes an exaggerated behavioural reaction to trauma
   b   Describes the appropriate response of the tissues to trauma
   c   Is currently classified in terms of the chemical mediators involved in the reaction to a specific category of trauma
   d   Is treated with histamine
   e   Describes an amplified and inappropriate inflammatory response of the tissues to physical or chemical trauma

3 The type I hypersensitivity reaction:
   a   Is mediated principally by IgG antibodies
   b   Provokes a widespread release of histidine from mast cells
   c   Causes a potentially fatal increase in blood pressure
   d   Results from a reaction between an allergen and a pre-existing IgE antibody

4 Tissue and organ responses to the type I reaction include:
   a   Urticaria
   b   Hypertension
   c   Diarrhoea
   d   Mental depression
   e   Halitosis

5 Haemolytic disease of the newborn is caused by:
   a   A defect of fetal haemoglobin
   b   Antigen–antibody reactions due to Rh+ second baby and Rh− mother

   c   Phagocytosis of NK cells

   d   Placental allergens

   e   Anti-D immunoglobulins

6 TNF-α's primary role is concerned with:

   a   Interleukin turnover

   b   The regulation of cell survival

   c   Inhibition of apoptosis

   d   Enhancement of viral proliferation

   e   Dampening of the immune response

7 How does adalimumab block the inflammation of rheumatoid arthritis?

   a   It activates the cyclooxygenase enzyme

   b   By blocking the biosynthesis of inflammatory interleukins

   c   By competing with TNF-α at its receptor sites

   d   It intercalates in nuclear double-stranded DNA

   e   By enhancing the release of IL-1 from mast cells

8 Chemokines are:

   a   Important blockers of inflammatory peptides

   b   Chemoattractant peptides and proteins

   c   Chemorepellent fatty acids

   d   Inflammatory enzymes

   e   Inhibitors of wound healing

9 The clinical significance of the chemokines includes:

   a   An important role in metastasis

   b   Inhibition of cell recruitment

   c   Blocking lymphoid trafficking

   d   Inhibition of wound healing

10 The interferons:

   a   Are antibacterial chemokines

   b   Deactivate macrophages

   c   Enhance presentation of endogenous antigens to B cells

   d   Are strongly oncogenic

   e   Include useful antiviral agents

11 Clinical uses of the interferons include:

   a   Use as an adjunct to surgery for malignant melanoma

   b   Treatment of delayed wound healing

   c   Inhibition of T-cell toxicity

   d   Enhancement of B-cell proliferation

   e   Downregulation of TGF-β_1

Further reading

Caruso R, Sarra M, Stoifi C et al. Interleukin-25 inhibits interleukin-12 production and TH1 cell-driven inflammation in the gut. Gastroenterology 2009; 136: 2270–9.

Chen L, Zhang C, Wang Y et al. Development of autoimmunity in IL-14α-transgenic mice. J Immunol 2006; 177: 5676–86.

Cho M, Jung YO, Kim KW et al. IL-17 induces the production of IL-16 in rheumatoid arthritis. Exp Mol Med 2008; 40: 237–45.

Commins S, Steinke JW, Borish L. The extended IL-10 superfamily; Il-10, IL-19, IL-20, IL-22, IL-24, IL-26, IL-28, and IL-29. J Allergy Clin Immunol 2008; 121: 1108–11.

Croft M. The role of TNF superfamilies in T-cell function and diseases. Nature Rev Immunol 2009; 9: 271–85.

Dempsey PW, Doyle SE, He JQ, Cheng G. The signalling adaptors and pathways activated by TNF superfamily. Cytokine Growth Factor Rev 2003; 14: 193–209.

Ford R, Tamayo A, Keyi N et al. Identification of B-cell growth factors (interleukin-14; high molecular weight-B-cell growth factors) in effusion fluid from patients with aggressive B-cell lymphomas. Blood 1995; 86: 283–93.

Foster PS, Mattes J. IL-21 comes of age. Immunol Cell Biol 2009; 87: 359–60.

Hartl D, Latzin P, Marcos V et al. Cleavage of CXCR1 on neutrophils disables bacterial killing in cystic fibrosis lung disease. Nature Med 2007; 13: 1423–30.

Koenders MI, Joosten LAB, van den Berg WB. Potential new targets in arthritis therapy: interleukin (IL)-17 and its relation to tumour necrosis factor and IL-1 in experimental arthritis. Ann Rheum Dis 2006; 65(suppl 3): iii29–33.

Koh SJ, Jang Y, Hyun YJ et al. Interleukin-6 (IL-6) -5726C- promoter polymorphism is associated with type 2 diabetes. Clin Endocrinol 2009; 70: 238–44.

Langrish CL, Chen Y, Blumenschein WM et al. IL-23 drives a pathogenic T cell population that induces autoimmune inflammation. J Exp Med 2005; 201: 233–40.

Leca L, Laftavi M, Shen L et al. Regulation of human interleukin-14 transcription in vitro and in vivo after renal transplantation. Transplantation 2008; 86: 336–41.

Locksley RM, Killeen N, Lenardo MJ. The TNF and TNF receptor superfamilies: integrating mammalian biology. Cell 2001; 104: 487–501.

Menkhorst E, Salamonsen L, Robb L, Dimitriadis E. IL11 antagonist inhibits uterine stromal differentiation, causing pregnancy failure in mice. Biol Reprod 2009; 80: 920–7.

Quin LS. Interleukin-15: A muscle-derived cytokine regulating fat-to-lean body composition. J Animal Sci 2008; 86: E75–83.

Rossi D, Zlotnick A. The biology of chemokines and their receptors. Annu Rev Immunol 2000; 18: 217–42.

Sakurai N, Kuroiwa T, Ikeuchi H et al. Expression of IL019 and its receptors in RA: potential role for synovial hyperplasia formation. Rheumatology (Oxford) 2008; 47: 815 20.

Schmitz J, Owyang A, Oldham E et al. IL-33, an interleukin-1-like cytokine that signals via the IL-1 receptor-related protein ST2 and induces T helper type 2-associated cytokines. Immunity 2005; 23: 479–90.

Sheppard P, Kindsvogel W, Xu W. IL-28, IL-29 and their class II cytokine receptor IL-28R. Nat Immunol 2002; 4: 63–8.

Smolen JS, Maini RN. Interleukin-6: A new therapeutic target. Arthr Res Therapy 2006; 8 (suppl 2): S5.

Stock P, Lombardy V, Kohlrautz V, Akbari OF. Induction of airway hyperreactivity by IL-25 is dependent on a subset of invariant NKT cells expressing IL-17Rβ. J Immunol 2009; 182: 5116–22.

Van Houlton J, Plater-Zyberk C, Tak PP. Interferon-β for treatment of rheumatoid arthritis? Arthr Res 2002; 4: 346–52.

Xue H, Gao L, Wu Y et al. The Il-16 gene polymorphism and the risk of the systemic lupus erythematosus. Clin Chim Acta 2009; 403: 223–5.

5

Autoimmunity and autoimmune diseases

Objectives:

- Define autoimmunity.
- Know some of the autoimmune diseases.
- Be able to provide relevant information on the importance of the thymus in autoimmune disease.
- Be able to give a brief outline of immunological intolerance.
- Know examples of autoimmune disease, the organs and tissues affected, the symptoms, and the antigens and autoantibodies implicated.
- Be able to expand the acronym ANCA.
- Explain immunological tolerance with a definition and theories of immunological tolerance.
- Know what is meant by low-level autoimmunity: triggers and mechanisms.
- Be ready to give examples of genes implicated in autoimmunity.
- Know some contributory factors, e.g. gender – the X-chromosome, hormonal factors, environment.
- Be able to give a brief outline of the MHC gene and autoimmunity.
- Briefly discuss transplant rejection.

Autoimmunity

Autoimmunity may be defined as the inability of an individual organism to recognise an integral part of itself as self. The consequence of this may be the spontaneous initiation of an immune response in the form of an attack by the immune system on these cells, tissues or organs. The immune system generates autoantibodies directed at the body's own tissues, e.g. anti-myelin basic protein in multiple sclerosis and anti-transglutaminase in coeliac disease. The resultant pathological disorder is termed an 'autoimmune disease'; many have been identified and the list is still growing. Examples of autoimmune disease include Addison's disease, Crohn's disease, rheumatoid arthritis (RA) and systemic lupus erythematosus (SLE), and a fuller (but not comprehensive) list is given below.

Thymus development and autoimmunity

The importance of the thymus in autoimmune disease was illustrated by the experimental thymectomy of 3-day-old mice, which subsequently developed the symptoms of autoimmune disease, associated with a depletion of CD4+, CD25+, regulatory T cells. The thymus plays a crucial role in the normal development of effective cellular immune systems, and for repair of immune function after damage to the immune system. Myasthenia gravis provides possibly the most graphic illustration of the importance of a normally functional thymus for the prevention of autoimmune reactions. There is also some evidence for abnormal thymus function, histology and size with respect to SLE and thyrotoxicosis.

The traditional approach to the treatment of autoimmune diseases, e.g. RA and Crohn's disease, has been the use of anti-inflammatory agents such as high-dose corticosteroids, which attenuate the inflammatory reactions produced by autoimmunity, but which are associated with severe adverse effects when used routinely.

Newer strategies have now emerged, due mainly to advances in our knowledge of the mechanisms of the immune response coupled with the development of recombinant DNA technology. Essentially, the healthy immune system effectively recognises foreign invaders, e.g. organisms and cells, as foreign and destroys them, and is able to recognise what is 'self' and leave it to operate normally. An immense effort is being put into the identification of the factors and molecular mechanisms whereby the host is able to recognise and respond fast and effectively to foreign material and render it harmless, and to the identification of those that enable the immune system to recognise and spare that which is self. The phenomenon has been termed 'immunological tolerance', which prevents the immune system from attacking members of its host systems.

Clearly, knowledge of the mechanisms of immunological tolerance is important if the mechanisms of autoimmune disease are to be understood and the disease treated and, hopefully, cured (Table 5.1). Once the point(s) of failure within the immune system to recognise and spare self are identified, it will then be possible to approach rationally the treatment of autoimmune diseases.

Table 5.1 Tissues. Lesions and immune system mediators in some autoimmune diseases			
Autoimmune disease	**Tissue/organ**	**Lesions/symptoms**	**Antigens, autoantibodies implicated**
Addison's disease	Adrenal cortex	Adrenocortical insufficiency	Often antibodies against the enzyme 21-hydroxylase
Antiphospholipid antibody syndrome, also known as Hughes' syndrome	Blood	Coagulation	Lupus anticoagulant; anticardiolipin antibodies; *MTHFR*[a] mutation
Autoimmune hepatitis types AIH-1 and AIH-2	Liver	Liver inflammation and necrosis	[b]Type AIH-1: smooth muscle autoantibodies (SMAs) and/or antinuclear antibodies (ANAs); antibodies against soluble liver or pancreas antigens; type AH2: autoantibodies against, for example, liver + kidney microsomal antigens
Coeliac disease	Small intestine	Microvilli damage and inflammation; impaired absorption from lumen	Tissue transglutaminase autoantibody (tTGAb)
Endometriosis	Uterus; endometrium	Inflammation; miscarriage	Anti-laminin-1 autoantibody
Graves' disease	Thyroid gland	Hyperthyroidism; abnormally large secretion of thyroid hormones	Thyroid-stimulating antibodies, which stimulate TSH receptors on thyroid, leading to hyperthyroidism and goitre
Multiple sclerosis	Myelin sheath	Myelin sheath destruction	Myelin/oligodendrocyte glycoprotein
Myasthenia gravis	Neuromuscular junction	Muscle weakness	Autoantibodies to the nicotinic acetylcholine receptor
Psoriasis	Skin, joints (psoriatic psoriasis)	Scaly, dry skin with uncontrolled skin production; inflamed painful joints	Anti-calpastatin autoantibody
Rheumatoid arthritis	Inflammatory systemic disease	Painful, inflamed joints; affects mainly joints; destroys articular cartilage; may attack other tissues including lungs	Rheumatoid factor[c]; anti-citrullated protein/peptide antibodies

(continued overleaf)

Table 5.1 *Continued*

Scleroderma: two forms:			
Localised (morphoea)	Affects mainly skin	Thickening and coarsening of skin	
Systemic scleroderma	Skin; vascular tissues; internal organs	Thickening and coarsening of skin; apoptotic changes to internal organs; collagen laid down; may be rapidly fatal	Anti-centromere antibodies (ACAs); anti-Scl-70 antibodies
Vasculitis	Mainly blood vessels	Inflammation and destruction of vascular tissue due to migration of leukocytes	Anti-neutrophil cytoplasmic antibodies (ANCAs) – see text

[a] Methylenetetrahydrofolate reductase.
[b] Not comprehensive.
[c] Not specific to rheumatoid arthritis.
TSH, thyroid-stimulating hormone.

Vasculitis as a paradigm of autoimmune disease investigation, and rationale for identification of possible targets for biological drugs

'Autoimmune vasculitis' is the term given for inflammation of blood vessels due to an autoimmune attack by white blood cells of the blood vessel walls causing inflammation of the endothelial cell. Vasculitis can also be caused by infection, e.g. through *Staphylococcus aureus*. Autoimmune vasculitis is also termed 'ANCA vasculitis'. ANCA is the acronym for anti-neutrophil cytoplasmic autoantibody. These antibodies are mainly immunoglobulin G (IgG) and occur in monocytes and the cytoplasm of neutrophil granulocytes, which normally attack invading bacteria and viruses. The organs and tissues attacked by the immune system vary with the individual and with the form of ANCA present. ANCA glomerulonephritis (renal limited vasculitis), for example, attacks the kidneys selectively; Wegener's granulomatosis, which can affect a wide range of tissues, lungs, kidneys and the nasal passages, may not be correctly diagnosed initially and may be ultimately fatal if not treated. The factors responsible for the development of ANCA in neutrophils are unknown; there may be a genetic component.

The nature of ANCA

Three forms of ANCA have been identified, through their staining of ethanol-fixed neutrophils: cytoplasmic or classic (c)-ANCA, perinuclear (p)-ANCA and x-ANCA; c-ANCA stains throughout the granular cytoplasm of the neutrophil, whereas the more positively charged p-ANCA is drawn to the negatively charged nucleus; x-ANCA is a common feature of inflammatory bowel disease. The role, if any, of ANCA in autoimmune disease is not known with certainty. It may be causative or a cellular product of the autoimmune reaction. It is clear that ANCA-associated small vessel vasculitis can be fatal, which is consistent with a possible role for ANCA in the autoimmune attack on the tissues.

It appears that ANCA molecules with specificity for a membrane protein-ase, PR3, are critical in the development of vasculitis. PR3 protein is expressed in a subset of the PR3 family. Also, it has been found that the NB1 receptor mediates PR3 expression on neutrophils.

The autoimmune response of the neutrophil appears to be initiated by a cell surface receptor, the NB1 receptor. This receptor, when activated, initiates the expression of an autoantigen on the cell surface, and this reaction initiates the autoimmune reaction. It has been suggested that the NB1 receptor may therefore be a target for treatment of ANCA-associated vasculitis.

Treatment of vasculitis

The main objective of treatment is the suppression of autoimmune reactivity. Traditional treatments included prednisolone, a corticosteroid and metho-trexate, an antifolate and antimetabolite. Newer treatments aim to do the following:

- Block the action of tumour necrosis factor α (TNF-α),
  e.g. etanercept and infliximab (see page 96); these are examples of the newer biological drugs.
- Block β-cell action, e.g. rituximab (see page 97).
- Deoxyspergualin: this is a newer, as yet unlicensed,
  immunosuppressive drug in the UK (at the time of writing).
  It is a synthetic analogue of spergualin, which is a product of a bacterium,
  Bacillus laterosporus. It appears to target T-lymphocyte maturation
  and B-cell differentiation. It has been used in patients with refractory
  ANCA-associated systemic vasculitis with encouraging results
  (see below).

Immunological tolerance

Definition

The host immune system is ignorant of its own self-antigens and therefore does not react to them.

Theories of immunological tolerance

Several theories of immunological tolerance have been advanced to explain how the immune system ignores 'self-antigens':

- The clonal ignorance theory: the immune system ignores self-antigens; a self-antigen is any part of the organism that is capable, under certain circumstances, of provoking an immune response within that organism.
- The clonal anergy theory: the host immune system fails to respond to an antigen due to a failure of T or B cells to respond to the antigen.
- The regulatory T-cell theory: this theory suggests that T lymphocytes temper the intensity of autoreactive immune responses.
- The clonal deletion theory: also called acquired immunological tolerance, whereby the body destroys potentially self-reactive lymphoid cells during the development of the immune system.
- The ideotype network theory, which postulates the occurrence within the immune system of a battery of antibodies specifically directed against any self-reactive antibodies.

It is possible that immunological tolerance involves several, if not all, of these postulated mechanisms. It is also possible that the loss of immunological tolerance plays a not insignificant role in the aetiology of autoimmune diseases.

Low-level autoimmunity

Paradoxically, autoimmunity is not necessarily a bad thing and is now considered to be a normal component of the immune system when it operates at the appropriate level. This so-called low-level autoimmunity may be triggered during the early stages of an infection before damaging levels of an invading pathogen become harmful to the host. During the early stages of an infection, when relatively few pathogenic organisms are present, a protective immunological response may be initiated before invading antigens have built up a sufficient concentration to trigger the immune system's antibody response. Furthermore, low-level autoimmunity may detect neoplastic cells through the immune system's CD8+ T cells, thus blocking further neoplastic growth.

Triggers and mechanisms of autoimmune reactions

As discussed above, an appropriate level of autoimmunity may be important for the maintenance of a healthy organism. A critically important question is that which asks what factors generate inappropriate and self-harming attacks by the immune system on cells and tissues previously recognised as self. The factors and mechanisms that initiate and sustain autoimmune reactions and cause them to become chronic are, at the time of writing, unclear and the subject of intensive research.

Currently, several possible contributory factors have been identified, as follows:

- genetic factors
- gender
- hormonal factors
- environment.

Genetic factors

The relative immensity of the human genome complicates attempts to identify genetic sources of autoimmunity, as does the undoubtedly complex input of several genes in the aetiology of autoimmunity. Nevertheless, several single nucleotide polymorphisms (SNPs) have been identified through large-scale investigations, termed 'genome-wide association studies' (GWASs). A fundamental observation from GWASs is that genetic factors linked to autoimmunity are not necessarily specific to a particular autoimmune disease, e.g. it has been found that an allele of the gene encoding the interleukin IL-23 receptor (3'UTR C2370A) has been reported to be associated with, for example, psoriasis and relapsing–remitting multiple sclerosis, and there is evidence that the IL-23 receptor may also be a major susceptibility gene for Graves' ophthalmopathy. Similarly, it has been reported that the gene encoding interferon regulatory factor 5 (IRF5) is associated with SLE, inflammatory bowel disease and RA.

Other genes currently suspected of being causative or involved in autoimmune diseases are those responsible for the expression of the major histocompatibility complex (MHC), the immunoglobulins and the T-cell receptors. Immunoglobulins and T-cell receptors are important in the recognition of antigens and, as they have inherent variability, could and probably do give rise to lymphocytes that may be self-reactive, i.e. react to their host organism. There is also evidence that some MHC class II allotypes are involved in the aetiology of autoimmune diseases. HLA-DR2, for example, has been convincingly correlated with SLE and multiple sclerosis.

Epidemiological studies of genetic factors in autoimmune disease also strengthen the case for an important genetic component, e.g. in studies of the occurrence of the autoimmune diseases RA, SLE, type 1 diabetes and multiple sclerosis in monozygotic (identical) twins, disease concordance was four times higher than in dizygotic twins (see below).

Gender

It is clear that in many, if not most, cases, girls and women are more prone to autoimmune diseases than boys and men, e.g. the ratio females:males for SLE is 9 : 1, for RA 3.5–4 : 1 and for primary biliary cirrhosis 10 : 1. For Sjögren's syndrome, the differential is highest, ranging from around 9–20 females to 1 male. The reasons for this are unknown, although estradiol may be a very important contributory factor. Pregnancy provides anecdotal evidence for endocrine involvement in the aetiology of RA, because many women report a marked remission of RA symptoms during pregnancy.

The X-chromosome and autoimmunity

X-chromosome abnormalities have been implicated in the aetiology of auto-immune diseases, in particular the phenomenon of skewed X-chromosome inactivation. Normally, during the days after fertilisation, one of the X-chromosomes is randomly 'chosen' by the cell and largely silenced, i.e. will not be able to express most of the genes that it carries. The chromosome may originate from the male or the female gamete. Interestingly, the daughter cells 'remember' which of the two X-chromosomes was silenced. Normally, distribution is stochastic, i.e. governed by chance, and most females will be mosaics, having an approximately equal amount of male- and female-derived inactive X-chromosomes. Some females, however, due to, for example, mutations of the genes, or perhaps purely through chance, have a skewed X-chromosome distribution, where one cell type predominates, biased towards either the female or the male donor. It is possible to detect and measure skewed X-chromosome inactivation using the technique of X-inactivation analysis.

It should be remembered that skewed X-chromosome inactivation does not necessarily result in autoimmune disease. A problem is more likely to arise if the individual has a mutated gene that is expressed in a significantly high proportion of a certain cell type, e.g. in muscle, joints or the gastrointestinal tract; it has been reported that patients with severe invasive ovarian cancer had a significantly higher prevalence of skewed X-chromosome inactivation than healthy or borderline patients. This was done by selective digestion of the active X-chromosome only, followed by polymerase chain reaction (PCR) to amplify the CAG repeat of the androgen receptor gene on the inactive X-chromosome; this repeat is highly polymorphic (several variations). X inactivation was considered skewed if 90% or more of the cells preferentially used one X-chromosome.

Hormonal factors

Clinical observations suggest that hormonal changes may trigger autoimmune disease in some individuals, e.g. the onset of SLE in some girls at puberty, when oestrogen levels start to rise. The ratio of the incidence of SLE in female and male patients is approximately 10 : 1. Research into the effects of oestro-gens on immune function may provide novel treatments for the control of

SLE. Autoimmune disease might be precipitated as a result of, for example, microbial infection or through adverse maternal reaction to the presence of fetal blood cells in the maternal circulation.

Environment

This area is controversial, although there are reports that the environment, and particularly attention to hygiene, might influence the tendency to auto-immune disease, e.g. it is now generally accepted that there is a causative relationship between cigarette smoking and the severity and incidence of, for example, multiple sclerosis, RA, SLE, Graves' disease hyperthyroidism and primary biliary cirrhosis.

Infection can trigger autoimmune disease, e.g. patients may develop:

- rheumatic fever after a streptococcal infection
  (unknown HLA association)
- type 1 diabetes mellitus after viral infections, e.g. Coxsackie A or B virus, rubella or echoviruses (associations: HLA-DR4, HLA-DO2, HLA-DO8)
- reactive arthritis after, for example, infections with *Campylobacter*, *Salmonella*, *Shigella* or *Yersinia* spp.

Some cellular mechanisms implicated in loss of self-tolerance and onset and maintenance of autoimmune states

- Rogue behaviour of certain MHC genotypes, e.g. abnormal level of presentation of MHC-expressed self-antigens (e.g. self-peptides) to T cells, without induction of tolerance to the peptide.
- Failure of development of anergy (loss or reduction of responsiveness to an immunological challenge).
- Failure of FAS-mediated apoptosis of anergic B cells after secondary encounter with a CD4 T cell.

The MHC and autoimmunity

The MHC is situated on chromosome 6 in humans and is possibly the most important determinant of autoimmunity; it is also an important determinant of transplant rejection. The MHC has 140 genes, at least half of which are known to be involved critically in the functions of the immune system. The MHC genes are functionally subdivided into three classes, namely I, II and III. MHC genes may have alleles that express a peptide identified by the host immune system as foreign, thus initiating and sustaining an autoimmune response.

Nevertheless, not all the genes and their products implicated in autoimmune disease belong to the MHC complex. For example:

- the complement genes that have been implicated in the aetiology of SLE
- the *PTPN22* phosphatase gene (expresses protein kinase phosphatase N22), in RA, type 1 diabetes mellitus and SLE
- single gene-mediated autoimmune diseases e.g.:
  - AIRE (autoimmune regulator on chromosome 21q22.3), implicated in, for example, Addison's disease and some other autoimmune endocrine disorders
  - ALPS (autoimmune lymphoproliferative syndrome), which is caused by persistence and accumulation of lymphocytes in the lymph nodes, which become engorged and swollen (lymphoadenopathy), and enlargement of the spleen (splenomegaly). The patient becomes anaemic due to destruction of erythrocytes (haemolytic anaemia). It is also termed 'Canale–Smith syndrome'. The disease is associated with mutations of the *FAS* gene, resulting in the production of double-negative T cells associated with impaired apoptosis of activated T cells
  - FoxP3 (Forkhead box protein 3), named after a gene originally described in *Drosophila* spp., encodes a transcription–repressor protein in the immune system. This gene is involved in the development of normal self-tolerance, and mutations of this gene may result in malfunctional regulatory CD4 cells. Vitiligo, a skin depigmentation problem, results from one of these mutations.

Transplant rejection

Transplant rejection is the failure of transplanted tissue to be accepted by the recipient, and is mediated by both humoral (chemical) and T-cell-mediated reactions by the host immune system. Traditionally, relatively non-specific treatments include anti-inflammatory corticosteroids, inhibitors of cellular proliferation, e.g. azathioprine, and blockers of interleukin (IL-2), e.g. sirolimus. There are now biological treatments to inhibit transplant rejection mechanisms.

Case scenario: Crohn's disease

James is a 27-year-old man who presents to his GP with bloody diarrhoea and mouth ulcers. He had noticed that his bowel habit had changed over a few months, with more regular and looser stools than before. This was occasionally accompanied by crampy abdominal pain, and he had noticed that he had lost a few kilograms in weight. The bleeding had started 1 week earlier, and was noticed as red blood mixed in with and coating the stools. The pain had also intensified in the left lower abdomen, and he had started feeling more tired than usual.

The GP examined James, and suspecting inflammatory bowel disease referred him to the gastroenterology department at the local hospital. They organised blood tests, which showed a mild anaemia and raised erythrocyte sedimentation rate (ESR), and he went on to have colonoscopy which showed an extensive area of inflammation in the sigmoid colon and proximal rectum. This area was biopsied and the histopathology confirmed Crohn's colitis.

James was treated with an oral preparation of mesalazine, a pro-drug of 5-aminosalicylic acid, and a course of oral steroids. Unfortunately, despite a prolonged course of steroids, the pain and bleeding continued and treatment was changed to oral azathioprine. This immunosuppressant drug was unsuccessful from the start, after James developed a series of hypersensitivity reactions including severe nausea, arthralgia and myalgia.

When James developed tonsillitis and was noted to have a reduced immune response the azathioprine was stopped. At this stage James had been unwell for 5 months, lost over 10 kg in weight, and had taken a considerable amount of time off work. The team decided to try infliximab treatment. This monoclonal antibody treatment was given as an intravenous infusion and James noticed an improvement in his symptoms within a few days of the first dose. Infliximab infusions are now given every 8 weeks, and James continues to be in complete remission, has returned to work and has started to regain the weight that he lost when unwell. He tolerates the infusions well, although gets an itchy rash.

Multiple choice questions

For each question, five options are provided and only one is correct.

1 Autoimmunity may be defined as:
   a   The ability of an organism to recognise a foreign protein as self
   b   The generation of antibodies to native proteins
   c   The immune system's inability to recognise an integral protein as self
   d   The automatic recognition by the immune system of foreign antigens
   e   An inherited immune response to a specific foreign antigen
2 Immunological tolerance may be defined as:
   a   The recognition of certain foreign proteins as self by the immune system

b   The ability of the host immune system to recognise and spare proteins of its own host

c   The mechanism whereby foreign metalloproteins are distinguished from those that are self

d   The failure of the host immune system to attack a virus or bacterium

e   The mechanism of action of certain antibacterial vaccines

3 Autoimmune vasculitis may be caused by:

a   Inflammation of epithelial cells of blood vessel walls

b   Retroviral infection

c   Staphylococcal infection

d   Liver inflammation

e   Hypothyroidism

4 ANCA is:

a   The acronym for anti-neutrophil cytotoxic antibody

b   An autoimmune disease of blood vessel walls

c   Caused by streptococcal infection

d   Characterised by inflammation of the epithelial lining of blood vessels

e   Mediated through IgM antibodies

5 ANCA is currently treated:

a   By blocking the action of IL-6

b   With α-adrenergic antagonists

c   With propranolol

d   With immunosuppressant drugs

e   By irradiation

6 Immunological tolerance occurs when:

a   The host immune system does not react when challenged by a foreign antigen

b   T and B cells fail to recognise the antigen

c   The patient ceases to respond to treatment with an anti-inflammatory antibody

d   The patient develops hyperlipidaemia

e   The body fails to destroy potentially self-reactive lymphoid cells during development of the immune system

Further reading

Birck R, Warnatz K, Lorenz HM *et al.* 15-Deoxyspergualin in patients with refractory ANCA-associated systemic vasculitis: a six-month open-label trial to evaluate safety and efficacy. *J Am Soc Nephrol* 2003; 14: 440–7.

Canale VC, Smith CH. Chronic lymphadenopathy simulating malignant lymphoma. *J Pediatr* 1967; 70: 891–9.

Chen S, Sawicka J, Betterle C *et al*. Autoantibodies to steroidogenic enzymes in autoimmune polyglandular syndrome, Addison's disease, and premature ovarian failure. *J Clin Endocrinol Metab* 2009; 81: 1871–6.

Cooper GS, Miller FW, Pandey JP. The role of genetic factors in autosomal disease: Implications for environmental research. *Environ Health Perspect* 1999; 107(suppl 5): 693–700.

Drappa J, Vaishnaw AK, Sullivan KE *et al*. *Fas* gene mutations in the Canale–Smith syndrome, an inherited lymphoproliferative disorder associated with autoimmunity. *N Engl J Med* 1996; 335: 1643–9.

Halonen M, Eskelin P, Myhre A-G *et al*. AIRE mutations and human leukocyte antigen phenotypes as determinants of the autoimmune polyendocrinopathy-candidiasis-ectodermal dystrophy phenotype. *J Clin Endocrinol Metab* 2002; 87: 2568–74.

Ho Khanh T, Reveille JD. The clinical relevance of autoantibodies in scleroderma. *Arthr Res Ther* 2003; 25: 80–93.

Karlson EW. Cigarette smoking and autoimmune disease: What can we learn from epidemiology? *Lupus* 2006; 15: 737–45.

Knudsen GP. Gender basis in autoimmune disease: X chromosome inactivation in women with multiple sclerosis. *J Neurol Sci* 2009; 286: 43–6.

Kojima A, Prehn RT. Genetic susceptibility to post-thymectomy autoimmune diseases in mice. *Immunogenetics* 1981; 14: 15–27.

Kristiansen M, Langerød A, Knudsen GP, Weber BL, Børresen-Dale A-L. Ørstavik KH. High frequency of skewed X inactivation in young breast cancer patients. *J Med Genet* 2002; 39: 30–3.

Matsushita Y, Shimada Y, Kawara S, Takehara A, Sato S. Autoantibodies directed against the protease inhibitor calpastatin in psoriasis. *Clin Exp Immunol* 2005; 139: 355–62.

Sakagucchi S. The origin of FOXP3-expressing CD4$^+$ regulatory T cells: thymus or periphery. *J Clin Invest* 2003; 112: 1310–12.

Zhernakova A, van Diemen CC, Wijmenga C. Detecting shared pathogenesis from the shared genetics of immune-related diseases. *Nat Rev Genet* 2009; 10: 43–55.

6

Treatment of rheumatoid arthritis and other inflammatory disorders with biological drugs

Objectives:

- Be able to give examples of inflammatory disease, notably rheumatoid arthritis (RA).
- Know the principal symptoms of rheumatoid arthritis, disease progression and consequences for the patient.
- Be aware of the important biological and environmental factors associated with and possibly contributory to the pathogenesis of RA.
- Know the clinical criteria for the diagnosis of RA and current aims of treatment.
- Be able to outline the treatment of RA with biological drugs.
- Know why methotrexate is used in RA.
- Know how biological drugs are administered.
- Know some adverse effects of biological drugs.
- Be familiar with the mechanism of action and uses of some anti-inflammatory biological drugs:
  - abatercept
  - adalimumab
  - anakinra
  - etanercept
  - infliximab
  - rituximab.

Several inflammatory diseases, including some of autoimmune aetiology, are either being treated with biological drugs or under clinical investigation with these drugs. A list of some of these diseases is given below and representative examples are dealt with in more detail:

- Alzheimer's disease
- arthritis
- asthma
- atherosclerosis
- Crohn's disease
- colitis
- dermatitis
- diverticulitis
- hepatitis
- irritable bowel syndrome (IBS)
- systemic lupus erythematosus (SLE)
- nephritis
- Parkinson's disease
- psoriasis
- ulcerative colitis.

Traditionally, many of these have been treated with drugs such as analgesics and corticosteroids for the symptoms of the disease. The advent of the biological remedies has now radically changed the approach to treatment, because these drugs not only provide relief from pain, but block the important endogenous mediators of inflammation, having analgesic and anti-inflammatory actions, and also possibly significantly slow the chronic process of tissue damage, thereby extending the useful life of the tissues, organs and joints.

Rheumatoid arthritis

The principal symptom of rheumatoid arthritis (RA) is inflammation of the joints. Inflammation may also occur in other tissues, including, for example, the heart, lungs, kidneys and pleura. The cause is currently unknown, but may involve climate, working conditions and gender, because it is more prevalent in women (F:M approximately 2.5 : 1.0). RA is diagnosed through its distinctive effects on the joints and in skin, and the diagnosis is reinforced by the presence in serum of the rheumatoid factor (RF), although its presence is not mandatory for diagnosis of RA. RA is systemic in that it may attack several different joints, and in many cases appears to affect different joints at different times, hence the term 'migratory or flitting polyarthritis' used by some authorities. Over time, irreparable damage is done to the joint due to inflammation of the synovial membrane, which forms the lining of the tendon sheaths and the joints. As the disease progresses, it destroys the joint tissues and reduces joint mobility through, for example, erosion and tethering of the tendons. This means that the tendon becomes fixed to adjacent tissues, which restricts its movement. Eventually, use of joints in the hands and limbs is lost, and fingers and toes may become severely deformed. In the skin, subcutaneous nodules form, and vasculitis may also be diagnosed, which is the chronic destruction of blood vessels. Several other haematological, radiological and biochemical tests are used to confirm the diagnosis but are not dealt with here. RA has traditionally been associated with morbidity and significantly earlier mortality.

Important environmental and biological factors associated with or possibly contributory to the pathogenesis of RA

- Cigarette smoking.
- Tumour necrosis factor (TNF)-α activity.
- Abnormal and inappropriate B-lymphocyte activity, i.e. abnormal antibody production.
- Detection of circulating autoantibodies against Ig Fc; these autoantibodies have been termed 'rheumatoid factor', and they may be involved in the inappropriate presentation of antigens to T cells by B cells.
- Abnormal activity of certain signalling pathways in synovial tissue, e.g. the Wnt signalling pathway, which is involved in embryonic development and cell renewal. In patients with RA, it has been reported that the synovial cells have abnormally high activity of the *Wnt* gene, as well as a number of other genes for several of the cytokines, cell adhesion molecules and chemokines. At present, it is not known whether these abnormalities are causative or a result of the more fundamental abnormalities.

Diagnosis of rheumatoid arthritis – clinical criteria

The criteria listed below are those published by the American College of Rheumatology in 1987. Any four of the criteria listed below must be identified for positive diagnosis of RA:

- detection of serum RF
- morning stiffness for 1 hour or longer for 6 weeks or more
- arthritis in three or more joints persisting for 6 weeks or more
- persistence for 6 weeks or more of symmetrical arthritis
- persistence for 6 weeks or more of arthritis of the hand joints
- rheumatoid nodules
- observation, using hand radiographs, of changes, erosion or unequivocal bony decalcification.

More recently, The Royal College of Physicians published guidelines for management and treatment of RA in adults, which take into account the patient's history. In particular, these guidelines help to distinguish between RA and some other self-limiting inflammatory condition. For more information, the reader is referred to the publication by the Scottish Intercollegiate Guidelines Network *Management of Early Rheumatoid Arthritis* (see end of chapter).

Current aims of treatment of RA

- Slow the rate of disease progression.
- Control inflammation and pain; ideally the patients should be as free as possible from pain.
- Design the appropriate treatment regimen for each patient.
- Regular appointments with the clinic and the rheumatologist.
- Regular patient monitoring for adverse effects of treatments.
- Regular blood tests.
- Monitor patient compliance.

Treatment of rheumatoid arthritis with biological drugs

Traditionally, RA was treated symptomatically with non-steroidal and steroidal anti-inflammatory drugs, which still have a place in the management of RA. The use of these drugs is self-limiting through the corrosive effects of non-steroidal drugs such as aspirin on the gut and the serious effects of steroidal drugs on, for example, water retention and redistribution of body fat. Paracetamol is an alternative to aspirin for treatment of pain, but has a relatively low therapeutic index. Furthermore these treatments do not slow the progression of tissue damage and loss of hand use and mobility. Several drugs, e.g. methotrexate, penicillamine, gold and azathioprine, commonly known as DMARDs, or disease-modifying anti-rheumatic drugs, have been used for several years. These may provide symptomatic relief and slow the progression of the disease, but are associated with serious adverse effects and are relatively non-specific in their actions.

The biological DMARDs have been developed thanks to the advances made in molecular biology, and especially with regard to the identification of key cellular mediators of inflammation. Essentially, these are monoclonal antibodies (MAbs) directed against chemical mediators of inflammation, notably TNF-α, and interleukins IL-1 and IL-6. These MAbs compete with the endogenous ligands at their receptor sites on cells, e.g. CD20 and CD22, some of which have no identified endogenous ligand (at the time of writing).

The introduction of the biological drugs, also termed 'biological DMARDs', seems set to bring more benefit to patients in this respect but they too may have serious adverse effects due to the lowering of resistance to infection through their powerful inhibition of the immune system.

The advantages associated with the use of the new biological DMARDs include:

- Restoration of joint function and reduction in joint stiffness, swelling and pain
- Production of significant periods of remission from symptoms
- Significant extension of usable joint life
- Significant reduction of early morning stiffness of joints
- Measurable reduction of the rate of joint damage
- Measurable reduction of levels of measurable markers of disease, e.g.
  - ESR (erythrocyte sedimentation rate)
  - C-reactive protein
- Reduction in measurable disease activity scores.

Disadvantages

- A most serious consideration for prescribers and public health organisations such as the NHS is their current cost, which should, however, be mitigated through the considerable savings from reduced patient care costs associated with progressive disablement and severity of disease symptoms. Furthermore, with time the costs of these drugs should fall significantly.
- MAbs suppress the immune response and may facilitate opportunistic infections, which necessitates the careful screening of potential recipients for the presence of any potentially dangerous pathological condition, e.g. respiratory infection
- MAbs are contraindicated in patients with moderate-to-severe heart failure, active tuberculosis, known hypersensitivity to murine (mouse)-derived products (several biological DMARDs have murine-derived macromolecular components)
- Adverse reactions during and after administration (see below).

The use of methotrexate alone or together with biological DMARDs

Methotrexate is prescribed alone as a DMARD for RA. It does take down tissue swelling and reduces pain, and will slow the rate of progression of joint damage and degeneration. It is prescribed together with the biological DMARDs in order to attenuate any immune reaction to the latter. The drug needs to be used with caution because it is a folic acid antagonist, and it is recommended that a dose of 5 mg folic acid be taken with each weekly dose of methotrexate (usually 7.5–20 mg weekly). Regular blood cell counts are strongly recommended for patients who take methotrexate.

Administration of biological drugs

Many of the biological drugs, e.g. infliximab and rituximab, are administered by intravenous infusion and are therefore given under clinical supervision in hospital. A nurse, doctor or other carer, on the other hand, may administer etanercept to the patient in hospital or at home.

Intravenous infusion methods

Adverse effects of biological drugs

Adverse effects may be considered in terms of infusion-related reactions and post-infusion reactions, e.g. with infliximab, infusion-related adverse effects notably include dyspnoea, headache and urticaria. These effects cannot with certainty be attributed to the drug or the physical process of perfusion because, in at least one study, up to 40 of patients suffered adverse reactions to infusion of a placebo. Post-infusion adverse reactions with infused or injected TNF-α inhibitors include optic neuritis, central nervous system (CNS) demyelination and opportunistic malignancies, e.g. lymphomas. Adverse neurological reactions reported include seizures and the reader is advised to refer to the most up-to-date published data available for each biological drug. There is little doubt, however, that the introduction of the biological drugs, especially in the treatment of diseases such as RA, Crohn's disease and cancer (see Chapter 7), has vastly improved the quality and duration of life for many millions of sufferers of rheumatic diseases and cancer (see Chapter 7).

In principle, the biological treatments act in a manner similar to that of many of the more conventional drugs in that they are receptor-blocking drugs, which are designed to bind to specific cell surface receptors on, for example, T or B cells, thereby preventing the endogenous inflammatory agents from triggering the immune response. Examples are shown in Figure 6.1, and these are described in more detail here.

Abatacept

Abatacept (Orencia) is a soluble fusion protein, prepared by fusing the extra-cellular domain of the human cytotoxic T-lymphocyte-associated antigen (hCTLA-4) to a modified human G1 immunoglobulin. When abatacept binds to its target receptors, namely CD80 and CD86 on the T cell, it prevents endogenous ligands from binding and blocks the inflammatory cascade. Normally, two processes activate T cells, namely the binding of the T-cell receptor to the antigen–MHC complex on the antigen-presenting cell (APC) and the binding of the T cell's CD28 receptor to receptor proteins on the surface of the APC. Abatacept binds to the B7 protein receptor with high affinity and thus blocks binding of B7 protein, thereby blocking the

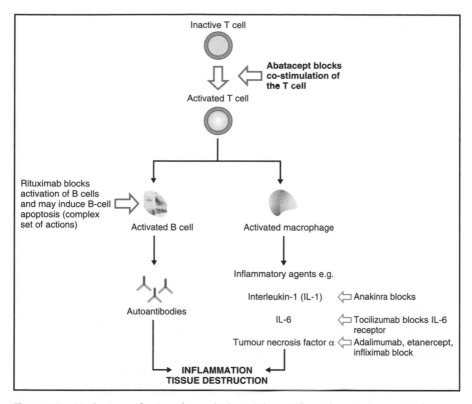

Figure 6.1 Mechanisms of action of some biological drugs. (After Cohen M. Abatacept in focus. *Internet J Rheumatol* 2007;**3**(1).)

inflammatory reaction. The site of action of abatacept on T cells gives it more scope as an immunosuppressant than others that act further down the inflammatory cascade, e.g. on the B cells.

Abatacept is prescribed together with methotrexate, another DMARD. This is because abatacept, as with the other biological DMARDs, is a foreign protein and may elicit an immune response by the host immune system. Methotrexate is a relatively small molecule that limits the immune response, thus sparing the foreign protein so that it can attenuate the host immune system's response.

Adalimumab

Adalimumab (Humira) is a completely human MAb that exhibits high affinity and specificity for TNF-α, blocking binding to its receptors. Adalimumab is supplied as a prefilled syringe containing 40 mg adalimumab, or as an auto-injector system and self-administered as a subcutaneous injection every other week. In some patients who do not respond satisfactorily to this dose it has been prescribed for once-weekly injection. It has been prescribed either alone or with methotrexate. It has been found to be effective not only for RA but also for Crohn's disease, (see below), ankylosing spondylitis and psoriatic arthritis. Patients usually feel the benefits about 1–4 weeks after starting treatment.

The adverse effects of adalimumab, as for many other biological drugs that block TNF-α, include susceptibility to opportunistic infections, including upper respiratory tract and urinary tract infections. Blood tests have revealed antinuclear antibodies (ANAs) in some patients with symptoms of SLE. Patients with latent TB may suffer reactivation during or after a course of adalimumab or with other biological DMARDs. Skin rashes, mouth ulcers and gastrointestinal disorders have been reported. Readers are referred to the *BNF* for more details of adverse reactions.

Anakinra

Anakinra (Kineret) is a recombinant antagonist at the IL-1 receptor. Chemically it is based on the structure of the IL-1RA receptor. It blocks the inflammatory actions of IL-1 by binding to it, thus blocking the cartilage degradation and inflammation caused by IL-1. In the UK anakinra is currently not recommended for the treatment of RA except as part of a clinical trial.

Etanercept

Etanercept (Enbrel) consists of a fully human amino acid sequence p75 TNFR11 dimer linked to the Fc of human IgG. It acts by blocking the binding of TNF-α to its receptor. It was the first biological approved by the US Food and Drug Administration (FDA) for the treatment of psoriatic arthritis. It is a dimer that can bind to two TNF-α receptors, whether free or cell bound, with very high affinity. As with several other MAb treatments, etanercept is often prescribed together with methotrexate. Through its widespread use, much is known of the clinical efficacy, safety and adverse effects of etanercept. The most frequently noticed adverse effect is a mild-to-moderate injection site reaction, which generally disappears with multiple use. The most serious adverse reactions, including fatalities, occur when the drug is used in patients who are also on immunosuppressant drugs, who are immunocompromised or who have existing infections such as sepsis.

Infliximab

Infliximab (Remicade) was the first biological anti-rheumatic treatment successfully developed for clinical use. It is a monoclonal antibody made up of a chimaeric human HgI–murine Fv1 gene complex, which binds both membrane-bound and soluble TNF-α with strong affinity. After infliximab administration, there are significant falls in the blood concentrations of some cytokines, notably IL1-RA (an IL-1 receptor antagonist), and of soluble TNF-α receptors, both of which contribute to the inflammatory response. These effects correlate well with the reduction in the symptoms of inflammation. Infliximab may also reduce the angiogenesis associated with the inflammatory response. Infliximab is still heavily prescribed in view of its high efficiency.

Rituximab

Rituximab (MabThera), together with methotrexate, is approved for the treatment of neoplastic diseases, e.g. follicular lymphoma (see page 70), and is also prescribed for RA in patients with active and severe RA that is refractory to other anti-rheumatic treatments. Rituximab was genetically engineered as a mouse/human chimaeric monoclonal IgG1 κ antibody directed against the CD20 receptor. It consists of variable light and heavy chain murine antibody sequences linked to constant human sequences. CD20 occurs as a transmembrane receptor on the surface of B cells and rituximab binds to it with very high affinity (molar dissociation constant about 7.5–10 nmol/L). Rituximab is administered by slow intravenous infusion.

The B cell clearly is a significant player in the aetiology of RA. In RA, the synovial cell B cells may secrete significant amounts of inflammatory cytokines including TNF-α. Furthermore, B cells may also function as APCs, which display the foreign antigen complex with the MHC on its surface. T cells may then recognise this complex through their T-cell receptor.

Clinical scenario – rheumatoid arthritis

A 14-year-old girl had presented initially at the age of 8 with painful flitting polyarthritis affecting mainly the hips, ankles, fingers and wrists. Radiographs revealed erosion in the ankles and hips, and throughout the history of her disease she had needed occasional use of a wheelchair. During flares she had been prescribed intra-articular steroid injections and infusions of methylprednisolone to extend remission periods. She was prescribed methotrexate at a dose of 17.5 mg once weekly and over the next 2 years was prescribed several different biological drugs, namely adalimumab, etanercept and infliximab. Eventually rituximab (1 g – a humanised anti-CD20 MAb) was prescribed by intravenous infusion with a repeated infusion of this dose after 2 weeks. Parameter changes: the Child Health Assessment Questionnaire (CHAQ) score dropped from 1.6 before treatment to 0.3 after treatment. Active joint counts were reduced from 6 to 0.

Psoriasis

Psoriasis is a chronic inflammatory disease that targets principally the skin and one that is possibly of autoimmune aetiology. Skin in many patients becomes reddened and scaly (psoriatic plaques) due to inflammatory reactions and excessive production of skin in these localised areas. There is no general pattern to the distribution of plaques and several forms have been identified. Plaques may occur, among other regions, on the legs and arms, at the joints, on the genital organs or on the scalp. These are the most prevalent forms and are termed 'psoriasis vulgaris' or 'plaque psoriasis'. In some patients inflammation is confined to finger- and toenails, when the term 'psoriatic nail dystrophy' is used. A form of arthritis (psoriatic arthritis) is diagnosed when the inflammation occurs at the joints. Other forms of psoriasis include flexural psoriasis, which manifests itself in the folds of the skin, e.g. under the arms or on genital folds. The most severe and potentially fatal form is erythrodermic psoriasis, when most of the skin peels off with consequent loss of temperature regulation and the loss of barriers to the external environment. In addition to physical stress, many patients with this (and other disfiguring skin conditions) become acutely self-conscious and may even become reclusive.

The cause or causes of psoriasis are unknown with certainty, and theories are based on the degree of success of different treatments, e.g. the success of immunosuppressants in temporarily clearing plaques lends weight to the idea that psoriasis may be an autoimmune disease. Alternatively, the lesion may be confined to the skin itself, in which there is abnormal and unregulated overproduction of skin in certain areas of the body. Dry as opposed to oily skin appears more vulnerable. Stress, infection or seasonal factors may contribute. Putative chemical irritants include alcohol, cigarette smoking and drugs, e.g. β blockers and chloroquine, an antimalarial drug. Precipitation of the disease has been reported following, for example, antimalarial drugs, antibiotics such as streptomycin, β blockers and lithium salts.

The genetic aetiology of psoriasis (and of course those of several other inflammatory diseases) is currently the subject of much research because this knowledge provides direction for the design of biological drugs. In the case of psoriasis, linkage analysis, which attempts to establish links between different genes in families in order to study disease-producing mutations, has produced evidence for at least nine loci on different chromosomes that are linked to the occurrence of psoriasis. The genes identified are called psoriasis susceptibility genes 1–9 (PSORS1–9). Several of these mutated genes have been implicated in the occurrence of psoriasis. An interesting finding is that gene PSORS1, on chromosome 9, which is the most commonly occurring linkage gene, controls the production of certain proteins that occur in abnormally high amounts in the skin of people with psoriasis, and also the production of components of the immune system. Of particular interest are genes that direct the upregulation of TNF-α and interferon-α.

Treatment of psoriasis

Traditional treatment may be topical, when soothing and emollient creams, lotions and ointments are applied directly to affected areas. Drugs used are relatively traditional preparations, including coal tar and mineral oil, and topical corticosteroids. These are of limited value, and corticosteroids are associated with skin thinning and rebound flares when withdrawn from use. Traditional systemic treatments include corticosteroids, which have severe adverse effects with prolonged use. Other immunosuppressants used include anti-metabolites and cytotoxic drugs, e.g. methotrexate, azathioprine and ciclosporin.

Treatment of psoriasis with biological drugs

The biological drugs used target specific inflammatory mediators or cells (see above). Drugs used include adalimumab, etanercept, infliximab and ustekinumab, which binds to IL-12 and IL-23 and blocks their action.

Systemic lupus erythematosus

SLE (lupus) is an autoimmune inflammatory disease that attacks mainly the connective tissues of the body. It may be localised to specific areas, organs and tissues, or be widespread. Tissues and organs commonly attacked include the heart, lungs, blood, skin, kidneys, liver and the nervous system. The disease is generally characterised by intermittent flare-ups and periods of remission. Gender plays an important part because the ratio of occurrence in women:men is about 9 : 1 and is more prevalent in non-European populations. Currently there is no known cure and SLE is treated symptomatically and in an attempt to blunt the immune system.

Aetiology of SLE

The cause or causes of SLE are unknown. Symptoms vary with the parts of the body affected. The common symptom is inflammation. It is not always easy to diagnose when symptoms first present themselves and may easily be misdiagnosed, e.g. a patient, perhaps a teenage girl, may soon after the onset of menstrual cycles start to exhibit aberrant and violent emotional behaviour, which may be dismissed as a sign of adolescence and if left untreated may result in a full-blown psychosis. This results from inflammation of the meninges or neuronal blood vessels. In other patients, the symptoms may include fatigue, joint pain and malaise.

A fairly definitive symptom is the malar or butterfly rash on the face. The skin is particularly susceptible, and patients may present with inflamed, scaly patches on the skin, referred to as discoid lupus. Mucous membranes are susceptible to the inflammatory reaction. Patients complain of ulcers of the vagina, mouth or nose. Alopecia (hair loss) may occur. More seriously, there may be inflammation of pulmonary tissues resulting in, for example, shrinking lung syndrome, pulmonary hypertension and pulmonary emboli.

Perhaps the most serious manifestation of lupus is in the kidneys, when the patient presents with painless proteinuria or haematuria. If left untreated this may result in acute or end-stage renal failure.

Crohn's disease

Crohn's disease is named after the American gastroenterologist Burril Bernard Crohn, although the diagnosis of inflammatory bowel disorders is historically well documented and the disease may be named according to the region of the bowel affected e.g. Crohn's ileitis, which is confined to the ileum, and the more prevalent type, which attacks mainly the large intestine. Crohn's disease affects both the ileum and the large intestine. Symptoms include fever and weight loss in adults and growth retardation in children. There may also be other symptoms, e.g. inflammation of other tissues including the skin and eyes. The disease predisposes some patients to the possibility of malignant growths in the areas affected. The causes of the disease are not known with certainty, but probably involve both environmental and genetic inputs. In contrast to the role of hyperimmune activity in, for example, SLE and RA, Crohn's disease appears to result from innate immune deficiency, possibly caused by a failure of macrophages to secrete certain protective cytokines. This exposes the patient to infection by opportunistic microorganisms. Patients generally experience periodic remission and relapse, and the aim of treatment is to sustain the periods of remission and prevent or diminish the damaging impact of relapse.

Diagnosis is confirmed using endoscopy, radiology and biopsy investigation.

Treatment is currently aimed at the treatment of symptoms when they occur and the establishment and maintenance of remission. Traditionally, glucocorticoids (corticosteroids) and 5-aminosalicylic acids have been used to treat inflammation and pain during relapse, and also immunosuppressant drugs such as methotrexate and azathioprine. More recently, newer biological drugs that inhibit the action of TNF-α, e.g. adalimumab and infliximab, are being used and these have proven, in many patients, to be very effective for inducing and maintaining remission.

More recently, it has been reported that naltrexone may be useful for induction and maintenance of remission.

The impact of treatment costs on treatment of RA (and other autoimmune problems) with biological drugs

The prevalence of RA is such that there is relatively heavy prescribing of the biological drugs, which at present are expensive when compared with the older treatments, e.g. a vial of infliximab (Remicade) was priced in the September 2009 issue of the *BNF* (*British National Formulary*) at £419.62 for a vial containing 100 mg. Assuming a patient weight of 65 kg, and given that the recommended dose is 3 mg/kg, the patient would be given 195 mg from two vials at a cost of £839.24. After 2 and 6 weeks the same doses are given, incurring a further cost of £1678.48, followed by similar doses every 8 weeks, which adds a further six treatments costing £5034.44. The total cost over 12 months is therefore £7552.16. In terms of patient relief from pain, improved quality of life and the slowing of the degenerative process, the cost becomes irrelevant. Furthermore, if previous experience is anything to go by, the cost of these treatments is likely to fall, particularly when generic alternatives become available.

Multiple choice questions

For each question, a maximum of five options is provided and only one is correct.

1 Factors possibly contributory to RA pathogenesis include:
 a Abnormally high TNF-α activity
 b Deficient antibody production
 c Mutations of rheumatoid factor
 d Abnormally low expression of the *Wnt* gene
 e Persistent hyperthermia

2 The clinical criteria for diagnosis of RA include:
 a Rheumatoid nodules
 b Absence of rheumatoid factor
 c Persistence for 7 days or more of morning stiffness for 1 hour or longer
 d Persistence for 2 weeks or more of arthritis in three or more joints
 e Raised white cell count

3 Current aims of treatment of rheumatoid arthritis:
 a Control of pain using sustained-release salicylate therapy
 b Three-weekly appointments with the district nurse
 c Slow the rate of disease progression
 d Regular counselling

---

4 The use of drugs to treat RA:

a   Salicylates no longer have a place in the management of RA

b   Paracetamol is not an alternative to aspirin for the treatment of pain

c   DMARD is the acronym for dental management with arthritis and other rheumatoid diseases

d   Biological drugs, including TNF-α antagonists, are now prescribed for the treatment of RA

e   MAbs have no place in the treatment of RA

5 Rituximab is an antineoplastic MAb, which:

a   Is not approved for the treatment of RA

b   Is directed against the CD18 receptor

c   Is a mouse/human chimaeric monoclonal IgG1 κ antibody

d   Is unavailable in the UK

e   Is administered by subcutaneous injection

Reference

Scottish Intercollegiate Guidelines Network. *Management of Early Rheumatoid Arthritis.* SIGN Publication No. 48. Edinburgh: SIGN, 2000.

Further reading

Arnett FC, Edworthy SM, Bloch DA *et al.* Revised criteria for the classification of rheumatoid arthritis. *Arthr Rheum* 1988; 31: 315–24.

Barton JL. Patient preferences and satisfaction in the treatment of rheumatoid arthritis with biologic therapy. *Patient Prefer Adherence* 2009; 3: 335–44.

Cohen M. Abatacept in focus. *Internet J Rheumatol* 2007; 3(1).

Edwards JCW, Szczepanski L, Szechinski J *et al.* Efficacy of B-cell targeted therapy with rituximab in patients with rheumatoid arthritis. *N Engl J Med* 2004; 350: 2572–81.

Genant HK, Peterfy CG, Westhovens R. Abatacept inhibits progression of structural damage in rheumatoid arthritis: results from the long-term extension of the AIM trial. *Ann Rheum Dis* 2008; 67: 1084–9.

Goffe B, Cather JC. Etanercept: An overview. *J Am Dermatol* 2003; 49(2S suppl): S105–11.

Kavanaugh A, Cohen S, Cush JJ. The evolving use of tumor necrosis factor inhibitors in rheumatoid arthritis. *J Rheumatol* 2004; 31: 1881–4.

Koenders MI, Joosten LAB, van den Berg WB. Potential new targets in arthritis therapy: interleukin (IL)-17 and its relation to tumour necrosis factor and IL-1 in experimental arthritis. *Ann Rheum Dis* 2006; 65(suppl iii): 29–33.

Kunz M. Current treatment of psoriasis with biologics. *Curr Drug Discov Technol* 2009; 6: 23–40.

Maini RN, Feldman M. How does infliximab work in rheumatoid arthritis? *Arthritis Res* 4 (suppl 2): S22–8.

Merck. Rheumatoid arthritis. *The Merck Manuals Online Medical Library.* Available at www.merck.com

Pincus T, O'Dell JR, Kremer JM. Combination therapy with disease-modifying antirheumatic drugs in rheumatoid arthritis: a preventive strategy. *Ann Intern Med* 1999; 131: 768–74.

Senolt L, Vencovsky J, Pavelka K *et al.* Prospective new biological therapies for rheumatoid arthritis. *Autoimmune Rev* 2009; 9: 102–7.

Smith JP, Stock H, Bingaman S, Mauger D, Rogosnitzky M, Zagon IS. Low-dose naltrexone therapy improves active Crohn's disease. *Am J Gastroenterol* 2007; 102: 820–8.

7

Development of biological antineoplastic drugs

Objectives:

- Have some knowledge of traditional forms of treatment for neoplastic disease.
- Be able to list important aims of the newer biological drugs.
- Describe and discuss mechanisms and targets for biological antineoplastic drugs.
- Be familiar with the central role of the epidermal growth factor (EGF) receptor in the aetiology of cancer.
- Have knowledge of some of the members of the erbB family of receptor protein kinases.
- Be able to give an account of the activation of the EGF receptor systems.
- Know some other ligands for the EGF receptor.
- Be able to give examples of biological antineoplastic drugs currently in use or development.
- Have some knowledge of precautions and responses to adverse reactions during treatment.

Traditionally, cancer has been treated symptomatically and with relatively non-specific cytotoxic drugs and inhibitors of cell division and protein synthesis. The introduction of the biological drugs enables prescribers to use the immune system to target specific components of the carcinoma and block their actions. The specific aims of the new drugs include:

- enhancing the immune system's ability to recognise and kill non-host cells
- enhancing the lethality of host immune cells
- blocking the mechanisms that turn benign host cells into cancer cells

- enhancing the host's ability to replace and/or repair host cells damaged or killed during the course of radiation or more traditional forms of non-specific cytotoxic chemotherapy.

Mechanisms and targets for biological antineoplastic drugs

Putative mechanisms that are potential or actual targets for antineoplastic drugs include:

- angiogenesis
- apoptosis
- cellular proliferation
- intracellular mechanisms, e.g. protein kinase activity
- metastasis
- molecular chaperones
- receptor activity and blockade
- transcription factors
- ubiquitin–proteasome pathways.

Cellular processes and biological molecules already successfully targeted by antineoplastic biological drugs include: (1) the epidermal growth factor receptor (EGFR), which is now targeted in the clinic by cetuximab and panitumumab; (2) HER2/neu (erbB-2), which is targeted by trastuzumab; and (3) the CD protein on B cells, which is targeted by rituximab.

The initial discovery that led eventually to the development of cetuximab and other drugs of similar action was that of the EGFR and its isolation and characterisation. The EGFR is a 170-kDa member of the family of erbB protein kinase receptors consisting of an extracellular ligand-binding domain, a transmembrane domain and an intracellular tyrosine kinase domain (Figure 7.1). The receptor also binds TGF-α (transforming growth factor α). Receptor activation promotes a number of cellular processes, including cellular differentiation, cellular mobility and cellular proliferation. Over-expression of EGFR-α is associated with a number of carcinogenic disorders, including bladder, colon, head and neck, breast and ovarian cancers. Furthermore, the EGFR may mutate and become carcinogenic.

The epidermal growth factor (EGF) is a polypeptide of molecular weight 133.1 kDa, and was originally isolated in extracts of mouse submaxillary glands as part of a much higher-molecular-weight complex, approximately 74 000. EGF is critically important for cellular differentiation, proliferation and survival of the cell. In the alimentary tract, EGF is essential for the maintenance of cell function, e.g. for protection of the mucosal surfaces from the corrosive actions of salivary, gastric and gastrointestinal tract secretions. EGF, in common with several other physiological mediators, forms part of a large group of structurally and functionally similar peptides and proteins

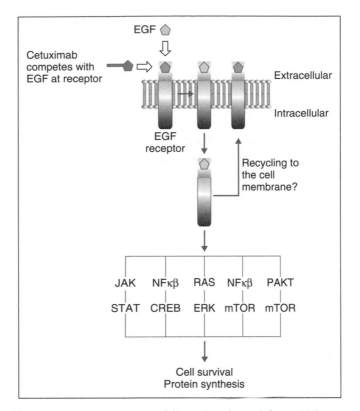

Figure 7.1 Diagrammatic representation of the epidermal growth factor (EGF) receptor. CREB, cAMP response element-binding protein.

called the neuregulins. Critically, for this chapter, EGF enhances cancer risk. For this reason, EGFR-blocking drugs are rapidly becoming an important treatment for cancer.

The EGFR family of tyrosine kinases

This receptor family is part of the erbB family of receptor protein kinases. Four genes encode these receptors:

- EGFR/*erbB-1*
- *c-erbB-2*/HER2
- *c-erbB-3*/HER3
- *c-erbB-4*/HER4.

The members of this family of receptors do not act in isolation when activated by the ligand, but work as an integrated system that ensures the appropriate cellular response to EGF. It is possible that, when one or more of these systems become unlinked from the system or become disabled, inappropriate cellular responses to EGF can result in a carcinogenic series of cellular reactions. The rationale of the modern anti-tumour necrosis factor (TNF) drugs is the blockade of these systems by blocking the receptors.

Activation of the EGF receptor systems

In the absence of EGF, the EGFRs reside on the cell surface in a quiescent state. When, however, EGF binds to its sites on the receptors, several interactive reactions and changes take place. Furthermore, the system comprises a complex mix of receptor types and ligands. Several ligands for EGF receptors have been identified, and termed members of an EGF receptor family, including:

- amphiregulin
- betacelullin
- EGF
- epigen
- epiregulin
- heparin-binding EGF (H-B EGF)
- neuregulins 1–4
- TGF-α.

Amphiregulin

Amphiregulin is a glycoprotein originally secreted from, among others, MCF (Michigan Cancer Foundation) cells and is also a member of the EGFR family. It has significant sequence homology with EGF and has strong affinity for EGFRs. Interestingly, it inhibits the growth of several different human tumour cell types *in vitro*, which raises the question about whether it may form one of a series of endogenous EGF-blocking or regulatory factors. As it may be involved in the regulation of EGF, it may play a role in normal tissue growth and modulate EGF action. It is known to be strongly proinflammatory.

Betacelullin

Betacellulin was initially isolated from an insulinoma cell line and stimulates DNA synthesis in, for example, vascular smooth muscle cells and fibroblasts. The highest concentrations have been found in the gastrointestinal tract and the pancreas. It does not appear to have angiogenic properties. It may function as a growth factor during cellular differentiation and organ development because it is expressed in endocrine precursors of the pancreas. It has also been detected in insulin-secreting cells in patients diagnosed with nesidioblastosis, a condition characterised by abnormally raised β-cell counts in the pancreas.

Epigen

Epigen (stands for epithelial mitogen) was originally identified through the sequencing of a mouse keratinocyte library and shows significant homology to the EGF family. Epigen is expressed mainly in the heart, liver and testis. When tested on epithelial cells *in vitro*, epigen stimulated phosphorylation of several kinase systems, e.g. mitogen-activated protein kinases and *c-erbB-1*, a growth factor receptor gene. It may also be a mitogen for cells that express several other growth factors.

Epiregulin

Epiregulin is an autocrine growth factor for human keratinocytes, and is a member of the EGF family. It was originally identified in medium from a culture of NIH-3T3 clone T7 cells, an epithelial mink lung cell line. Epiregulin is able to stimulate proliferation of human keratinocytes *in vitro* in the absence of EGF. It has a positive feedback action in that epiregulin upregulates levels of its own mRNA, as well as those of other EGF-like growth factors, e.g. mRNA of amphiregulin, H-B EGF-like growth factor and TGF-α. The system has a positive feedback mechanism since those factors in turn stimulate epiregulin mRNA synthesis.

Heparin-binding EGF

H-B EGF was originally discovered in conditioned medium from human macrophages. It has powerful chemotactic and mitogenic properties with regard to human macrophages. It stimulates proliferation of several different cell types, e.g. stromal cells, and has high affinity for at least two types of EGFR. It has also been shown to be a very powerful inducer of angiogenesis and tumour growth.

Neuregulins

The neuregulins are a group, or family as they are frequently called, of products of four genes, namely NRG-1, -2, -3 and -4. These genes all encode proteins with an EGF-like domain and activate erbB receptor kinases. They are critically important in, for example, development and oncogenesis. There is growing evidence that the neuregulin 1 (NRG1) type IV gene is an important susceptibility gene for schizophrenia. Specifically, the NRG1 locus on chromosome 8p exhibits linkage to schizophrenia. There is evidence that NRG1 is critically important in neuronal development and function. Specifically, it is involved in synaptogenesis, neuronal migration and glial development. Normal heart development is dependent on the normal functioning of NRG1. Experimental studies have shown that fetal mice lacking NRG1 do not have normal development of the cardiac trabeculae and do not survive. Neuregulin 3 (NRG3) appears to be critically important in the development and normal functioning of the nervous system. NRG4 is a growth factor with an mRNA that has been found mainly in the pancreas and weakly in muscle.

Many of the growth factors dealt with in this section are anchored to the cell membrane, and until activated exist in a nascent state. The unravelling of this complex system of ligands (and possibly antagonists) may provide yet more clinical tools in the search for specific and effective treatments for cancer.

Some biological antineoplastic drugs currently in use or development

This is a rapidly growing list (Table 7.1).

Alemtuzumab (MabCampath)

Alemtuzumab is a recombinant, humanised, DNA-derived, monoclonal antibody used to treat refractory chronic lymphocytic leukaemia. It binds to CD52, a cell surface receptor on virtually all B and T lymphocytes, certain granulocytes, monocytes and macrophages. This results in lysis of the leukaemia cells. It is supplied as a concentrated solution (30 mg/mL) and diluted as directed by the manufacturer immediately before being given as an intravenous infusion.

Bevacizumab (Avastin)

Bevacizumab is a humanised monoclonal antibody that binds the vascular endothelial growth factor receptor and blocks it. In the UK it is licensed to treat metastatic colorectal cancer together with fluoropyrimidine-based chemotherapy. It is also licensed to treat advanced or metastatic renal cell

Table 7.1 Some biological antineoplastic drugs

Drug	Target	Proprietary name	Therapeutic use
Bevacizumab	Vascular endothelial growth factor receptor (EGFR)	Avastin	Metastatic colorectal cancer
Cetuximab	EGFR inhibitor	Erbitux	Metastatic colorectal cancer/ squamous cell cancer of the head
Panitumumab	EGFR inhibitor	Vectibix	Metastatic colorectal cancer
Trastuzumab	Blocks HER2/neu receptor	Herceptin	Early breast cancer that over-expresses HER2

carcinoma together with interferon-α_{2a}, and for first-line treatment of metastatic breast cancer in combination with paclitaxel. It is administered as an intravenous infusion.

It is formulated as a 25 mg/mL concentrate for intravenous infusion.

Cetuximab (Erbitux)

This is formulated as 5 mg/mL solution for intravenous infusion (see below).

Erlotinib and gefitinib

Erlotinib (Tarceva)

Erlotinib is a relatively small molecule compared with the biological antibodies (M_r of approximately 393 g/mol). Its systematic IUPAC (International Union of Pure and Applied Chemistry) name is N-(3-ethynylphenyl)-6-7-bis(2-methoxyethoxy)quinoxolin-4-amine.

The mechanism of clinical antitumor action of erlotinib is not fully characterised. Erlotinib inhibits the intracellular phosphorylation of tyrosine kinase associated with the EGFR. Specificity of inhibition with regard to other tyrosine kinase receptors has not been fully characterised. EGFR is expressed on the cell surface of normal cells and cancer cells.

Effectiveness of the biological treatments for cancer

Lung cancer

Cetuximab as a paradigm of a biological drug for cancer treatment

Conceptually, the principal advances and procedures are:

- the identification of key mediators of cellular proliferation and of their receptors on the target cell, in this case EGF and EGFR
- the development of antagonists that block the binding of the mediator to its receptors
- the pharmaceutical formulation and clinical screening of the antagonist before the release of the drug for routine clinical use.

Formulation and activity

Cetuximab is a monoclonal antibody to the cell membrane EGFR and is able to block the binding of EGF to its receptor, thus blocking or attenuating its neoplastic actions. The cetuximab–EGFR complex is internalised and destroyed by the cell, thus also reducing the numbers of available EGFRs for recycling back to the membrane.

Cetuximab is formulated as a chimaeric mouse–human monoclonal antibody at a concentration of 5 mg/mL and the solution volume is 20 mL.

Indications for use

In the UK, cetuximab is licensed for the treatment of metastatic colon cancer in patients whose tumours are refractory to other treatments, and if the tumours express the EGFR. It is also licensed in patients who are intolerant to other treatments, e.g. it has been used in the following situations:

- together with radiotherapy for use in patients with locally advanced squamous cell tumours of the head and neck
- co-prescribed with irinotecan, a topoisomerase 1 inhibitor, particularly in patients with EGFR-expressing metastatic colorectal cancer
- together with radiation therapy for locally advanced disease states
- together with platinum-based chemotherapy for metastatic and or recurrent disease
- as a treatment for patients who cannot tolerate irinotecan, or who have failed irinotecan and oxaliplatin chemotherapy
- at the time of writing, the National Institute for Health and Clinical Excellence (NICE) has allowed the use of cetuximab for locally advanced squamous cell cancer of the head and neck.

It should be noted that trials of cetuximab together with irinotecan were reported to be ineffective in patients with *K-ras* mutations in codons 12 or 13 of the tumour. The *K-ras* gene is an oncogene, the mutations of which are of central importance in the development and progression of neoplastic disease, especially in colorectal, pancreatic and lung cancers.

Supply

Cetuximab is supplied in sterile, colourless liquid form at a pH of 7.0–7.4 and at a concentration of 5 mg/mL for infusion. Volumes supplied are 10, 20, 50 and 100 mL. Amorphous-looking particles of cetuximab may be visible in the vial.

Patient assessment before giving cetuximab (or any other monoclonal antibody)

Blood and urine samples must be taken and tested for evidence of infection and anaemia, including:

- platelet and leukocyte counts
- serum creatinine
- serum transaminase
- haemoglobin
- bilirubin
- any other parameters mentioned in manufacturer's literature.

Patients presenting with any symptoms suggesting that an infection is present must not be given a drug that can further weaken the immune system. In addition, patients require especially close monitoring during administration if there is a history of cardiovascular or pulmonary disease.

Preparation of cetuximab for administration

Preparation must be carried out under aseptic conditions and strictly in accordance with the manufacturer's instructions.

Premedication, dosage and administration

Cetuximab, in common with other macromolecular infused drugs, should be administered in an environment geared to rapid response to adverse reactions to the infusion, particularly to anaphylactic reactions, preferably a clinic or hospital. It should be noted that patients must be prescribed an antihistamine before infusion of cetuximab.

Dose and administration

Cetuximab is supplied in 20 or 100 mL vials at a concentration of 5 mg/mL and is prescribed for infusion once a week. The loading dose is 400 mg/m^2, which is infused over a period of 2 h, using an infusion pump and an in-line filter. Subsequent doses are 250 mg/m^2 infused over a period of 1 h. During preparation, the liquid should not be vigorously shaken or agitated, and it should not be diluted. The preparation may contain floccular matter and no attempts should be made to disperse or dissolve this.

During infusion

The patient should be monitored regularly for blood pressure, temperature and, after infusion, the patient should be observed for at least 1 h in case of post-infusion adverse reactions.

Precautions and appropriate responses to adverse reactions during infusion

These usually present during the first infusion and often within the first hour: shock, fever, chills, dyspnoea, syncope, hypersensitivity reactions, e.g. hypotension, urticaria, bronchoconstriction and hypotension.

After infusion, patients should be advised to report immediately any symptoms, feelings of giddiness, headache, skin reactions, itchiness or pain, especially at the injection site. Patients should be advised to take no herbal or over-the-counter medication during the course of treatment. Serum cations, particularly magnesium, potassium and calcium, should be monitored regularly up to 8 weeks after the last infusion (taking into account the half-life of cetuximab). In addition, patients should be advised to maintain normal and adequate fluid intake and diet. Patients may experience photophobia and should wear protective clothing. Cetuximab, in common with many similar preparations, is contraindicated during breast-feeding, which in any event must not be done during treatment or for at least 60 days after the last infusion of cetuximab. Patients should keep medical staff fully informed about planned pregnancies before initiation of treatment.

Case history

A 62-year-old woman with a history of primary carcinoma of the left breast presented with metastases to the right axillary lymph node. High-dose chemotherapy induced a modest response. Mastectomy was decided upon, with bilateral biopsies of the axillary lymph nodes. After 8 months the patient was found to have multiple lung metastases and was treated with six cycles of vindesine, an antimitotic vinca alkaloid, mitoxantrone, a type II topoisomerase inhibitor and fluorouracil, which is a pyrimidine alkaloid, and is a non-competitive inhibitor of thymidylate synthase. This cycle produced a partial remission. *HER2* gene product was tested for on primary tumour cells and a positive result obtained. Accordingly, trastuzumab, an anti-HER2 monoclonal antibody, was prescribed by intravenous infusion. The pulmonary lesions were removed 2 years after the first dose of trastuzumab and tested negative for cancer cells. There has been no relapse for 18 months since pulmonary resection.

Multiple choice questions

For each question, five options are provided and only one is correct.

1 Biological mechanisms that are potential or actual targets for antineoplastic agents include:
   a   Synaptic transmission
   b   Renal clearance
   c   Hepatic metabolism
   d   Angiogenesis
   e   Lipid deposition
2 Cellular processes and molecules already targeted by antineoplastic biological drugs include:
   a   The neuromuscular junction
   b   The epidermal growth factor receptor
   c   Hepatic gluconeogenesis
   d   Tyrosine hydroxylase
   e   Carbonic anhydrase
3 Epidermal growth factor is critically important for:
   a   Cellular differentiation
   b   Protection of the cell from carcinogens
   c   Temperature control

> d   Gluconeogenesis
> e   Appetite control
>
> **4** Amphiregulin:
>
> a   Is a fatty acid secreted by CD20 cells
> b   Is a glycoprotein secreted from, among others, MCF cells
> c   Has weak sequence homology with EGF
> d   Strongly promotes growth of several human tumour cell types *in vitro*
> e   Is weakly proinflammatory
>
> **5** Cetuximab:
>
> a   Is a monoclonal antibody directed against EGF
> b   Is not co-prescribed with irinotecan
> c   Is administered by injection
> d   Is not licensed for therapeutic use in the UK
> e   Is formulated as a chimaeric mouse–human monoclonal antibody directed against the EGFR

Further reading

Bazley LA, Gullick WJ. The epidermal growth factor receptor family. *Endocr Relat Cancer* 2005; 12: S17–S27.

Folprecht G, Lutz MP, Scffski P *et al.* Cetuximab and itinotecan/5-fluorouracil/folinic acid is a safe combination for the first-line treatment of patients with epidermal growth factor receptor expressing metastatic colorectal carcinoma. *Ann Oncol* 2006; 17: 450–6.

Gilmour LMR, Macleod KG, McCaig A *et al.* Neuregulin expression, function, and signalling in human ovarian cancer cells. *Clin Cancer Res* 2002; 8: 393–94.

Gullick WJ. Prevalence of aberrant expression of the epidermal growth factor receptor in human cancers. *Br Med Bull* 1991; 47: 87–98.

Harari D, Tzahar E, Shelly M *et al.* Neuregulin 4: a novel growth factor that acts through the Rrb-4 receptor tyrosine kinase. *Oncogene* 1991; 18: 2681–9.

Higashiyama S, Abraham JA, Miller J *et al.* Heparin-binding growth factor secreted by macrophage-like cells that is related to EGF. *Science* 1991; 251: 936–9.

Li Seno M, Yamada H, Kojima I. Betacellulin improves glucose metabolism by promoting conversion of intraislet precursor cells to β-cells in streptozotocin-treated mice. *Am J Physiol Metab* 2003; 285: E577–83.

Ongusaha P, Kwak JC, Zwible AJ *et al.* HB-EGF is a potent inducer of tumor growth and angiogenesis. *Cancer Res* 2004; 64: 5283–90.

Plowman CG, Green JM, McDonald VE *et al.* The amphiregulin gene encoded a novel epidermal growth factor-related protein with tumor-inhibitory activity. *Mol Cell Biol* 1990; 10: 1969–81.

Ring HZ, Chang H, Guilbot A *et al.* The human neuregulin-2 (NRG2) gene: cloning, mapping and evaluation as a candidate for the autosomal recessive form of Charcot-Marie-Tooth disease inked to 5q. *Hum Genet* 1999; 104: 326–32.

Shirakata Y, Komurasaki T, Toyoda HG *et al.* Epiregulin, a novel member of the epidermal growth factor family, is an autocrine growth factor in normal human keratinocyters. *J Biol Chem* 2000; 275: 5748–53.

Taylor JM, Mitchell WM, Cohen S. Characterization of the high molecular weight form of epidermal growth factor. *J Biol Chem* 1974; 249: 3198–203.

8

Stem cell therapy

Stem cell therapy is the use of stem cells to treat disease. Stem cells are cells that have the ability to differentiate into other cell types and have the ability to function normally according to the cell type that results. They are the progenitor cells of the embryonic blastocyst (Figure 8.1) that will differentiate into the cells of all the body's disparate systems. These are the cells of the embryonic ectoderm, endoderm and mesoderm. In some texts stem cells are called pluripotent cells.

The reader will doubtless be aware of the intense ethical debate over the use of the human embryo, and is referred to publications devoted to the matter.

Ever since cells were first seen under the microscope and their biological functions studied, attempts have been made to use them for therapeutic purposes with variable success. As far back as the nineteenth century scientists knew that cells can reproduce and unsuccessful attempts were made to treat patients with cells. The science of embryology began in earnest with the discovery that embryonic cells can mutate with regard to structure and function, and in the mid- and late twentieth century the possibility of using stem cells in medicine received a boost when McCulloch and Till (1961) developed techniques for identifying and studying cell differentiation and for successfully transplanting stem cells. A number of research groups, succeeded in isolating mouse embryonic stem cells, and James Thomson developed the first human embryonic stem cell lines in the late twentieth century (Thomson *et al.* 1998).

The next logical step was the manipulation of adult-sourced cell lines to see if these could be altered, and at the turn of the last century scientists found a way to produce, for example, liver and nervous tissue from bone marrow cells.

The nature of stem cells

Stem cells differ from all other cell types in their ability to reproduce and, given the appropriate circumstances, mutate into cells of very different function, and replenish themselves after tissue damage. They differ in their versatility and have been classified in terms of their range.

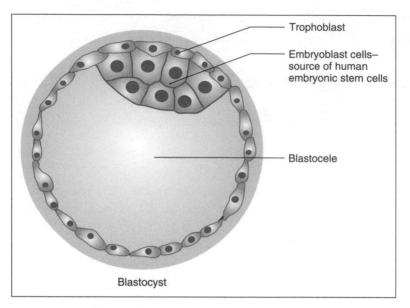

Figure 8.1   Embryonic stem cells.

Omnipotent/Totipotent

These cells are able to mutate into any other cell type in both an embryonic and extra-embryonic environment. The cells produced by the fusion of the female and male gametes are pluripotent; they will produce the complete new member of that species. The embryoblast cells of the blastocyst are therefore omnipotent.

Pluripotent

These are stem cell progeny of the omnipotent parent cell that can develop into cells of one of the three primary cell layers, i.e. the ectoderm, endoderm and mesoderm. The ectoderm cells, in vertebrates, are the outermost cell layer of the embryo and will develop into the epidermis, nervous system and sense organs of the fetus. The endoderm will develop into the digestive and respiratory systems. The mesoderm lies between the ectoderm and endoderm and will develop into, for example, bone, cartilage, circulatory system, connective tissue, gonads, lymph tissues and cells, and muscle.

Multipotent

These are more limited in scope for differentiation. They are the cells in the brain that will result in the neurons, glia and neuroglia. They cannot give rise to cell types other than that for which they are programmed. Bone marrow contains multipotent cells that can produce different species of blood cell, but cannot create, for example, neural cells.

Oligopotent

These cells are more limited in range in that they can mutate into even fewer forms of stem cells. Example include lymphoid and myeloid stem cells.

Unipotent stem cells

These cells can produce only one cell type; a skin cell is a classic example: it cannot become another cell type. It can, however, be the source of a seemingly endless supply of skin cell progeny.

Other properties of embryonic stem cells include the possession of a number of growth factors, notably Nanog, Oct4 and Sox2. The *Nanog* gene codes for a protein that maintains the property of pluripotency of the stem cell during cell culture. Oct4 (abbreviation of octamer-4) is a transcription factor the presence of which is also required to maintain the undifferentiated status of the embryonic cells. Sox2 is another transcription factor coded for by a sex-determining gene also termed Sox2 or SRY, with the same basic function as that of Oct4.

Embryonic stem cell cultures

Embryonic stem cell cultures are derived from the blastocyst (see above), and may also be derived from the earlier stage morula. The blastocyst may consist of about 100 cells on average. These cells are pluripotent, if not omnipotent, and can give rise to any of the three primary germ cell layers. Given the correct stimulation, these cells have the potential to give rise to any of the cells that make up the completely formed body. The placenta, incidentally, is not derived from these cells, but from the egg sac itself. Figure 8.1 is a diagram of an embryonic stem cell.

Preparation of stem cells from the blastocyst

After the blastocyst cells have been removed from the embryo, they can be grown on a feeder layer of murine (mouse) embryonic fibroblasts in the presence of basic fibroblast growth factor (bFGF) or fibroblast growth factor-2. Without this environment the embryonic cells would rapidly differentiate. After a period of incubation the cells are permitted to differentiate by culturing the cells and withholding the growth factors. During spontaneous differentiation they aggregate to form what is termed an

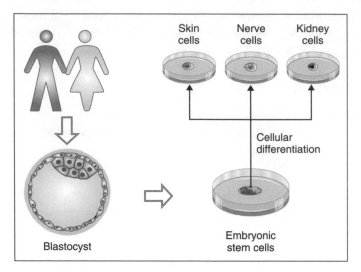

Figure 8.2   Embryonic stem cell production.

'embryoid body', and from it the cells of the ectoderm, endoderm and mesoderm are derived (Figure 8.2). The embryoid body develops initially as a layer of endoderm, then ectoderm and finally mesoderm. The embryoid bodies are incubated further and continue to differentiate into the different cell types of the body.

Adult stem cells

Adult stem cells are cells of the completely developed organism that have the ability to divide and duplicate themselves and mutate into another cell type. Examples include the following:

- endothelial stem cells
- haematopoietic stem cells of the bone marrow, which give rise to the cells of the blood
- mammary stem cells, which develop at puberty into the cells of the adult breast, and are also implicated in the development of carcinoma of the breast
- mesenchymal stem cells, which originate in stromal tissue, and have an important scaffolding role
- neural stem cells
- olfactory stem cells
- testicular stem cells.

Clinical use of stem cells

The clinical use of stem cells is, for most diseases, still in its infancy, although it is in use, notably for bone marrow transplantation. Important advances are being made – see the recent report of the growth and implantation of a human trachea from the stem cells of a patient (see below). The feasibility of bone marrow transplantation was first demonstrated as far back as the mid-twentieth century by E Donnall Thomas and his colleagues (Buckner *et al.* 1970), who initially reported in 1956 the intravenous infusion of bone marrow for patients undergoing chemotherapy and radiation, and went on to transplant bone marrow into a patient with leukaemia. Joseph E Murray, another pioneer of transplantation of tissues, performed the fist successful transplant of a kidney between monozygotic twins, and he and Thomas were jointly awarded the Nobel Prize for medicine in 1990. Today, thanks to advances in stem cell technology, bone marrow transplants have largely been replaced by haematopoietic stem cells harvested from human tissues, e.g. amniotic fluid, blood, bone marrow and umbilical cord blood.

As mentioned above, there has been an important development with the report on 23 March 2010 from Great Ormond Street Children's Hospital of the preparation and transplantation of a donor trachea transformed on a collagen-based scaffold and infused with stem cells from the patient.

Medical conditions for which stem are prescribed include aplastic anaemia, congenital neutropenia, AIDS, sickle cell disease, neuroblastoma and Hodgkin's disease.

Prospects and the future for regenerative medicine

For centuries, the philosophical bedrock of medicine has been the treatment of symptoms. Even now, with the advent of the newer biological therapies, the aim is to hold the symptoms at bay by blocking mediators of the disease. Now, with the development of stem cell technology, the aim of tissue and organ replacement is fast becoming a feasible alternative. Diseases hitherto relatively intractable to treatment can now be approached with a real expectation of symptom alleviation, and perhaps even a cure in some cases.

It is now feasible to envisage a branch of medicine in which cells can be harvested from patients and used to grow tissues, organs and perhaps even limbs to replace those lost through disease or injury. It has been estimated by the US Department of Health and Human Services that the worldwide market for regenerative medicine could soon reach a figure of around US$500 billion. Diseases such as type 2 diabetes, which is caused by a failing pancreas, or heart disease may in the not too distant future be curable through tissue and organ transplantation or regeneration.

At the time of writing, this is still a branch of medicine in its infancy, and only bone, cartilage and skin for clinical use have proven amenable to the available technology. Tools already in use include antibiotic bone filler, consisting mainly of polymethylmethacrylate and a radio-opaque additive such as barium sulphate or zirconium oxide, which has been used successfully to fuse artificial joints to the skeleton. Bone grafting, too, is the subject of much research. It is a necessary procedure for the successful treatment of certain forms of bone corrosion, whether from congenital defects or as a result of bone disease. It has been shown experimentally, using mice, that bone grafts can be vascularised by seeding the graft with bone-marrow-derived cytokines.

Another important advance will be the elucidation of the pathways to tissue renewal after damage, caused by, for example, ageing, pollution or injury. This is now an active research area, particularly with reference to the identification of adverse cellular conditions imposed on the injured or ageing cell, particularly those that cause damage to cellular DNA, especially in the stem cells. There is, for example a report that the *p53* tumour-suppressor gene is vital for the maintenance of tissue homoeostasis and the promotion of tissue renewal by limiting the accumulation of DNA-damaged cells.

It will also be necessary to focus on and develop a number of skills and methods if the list of available tissues is to be expanded. These include a greater understanding of the factors that dictate stem cell manipulation in order to direct the creation of specifically chosen tissues and organs. Clearly, there will have to be a greater emphasis on this research in both the academic and industrial sectors and adequate financial support. Much more has to be known about the chemical and physical reactions that underlie tissue–tissue interactions and influences on each other. The nuts and bolts of intercellular signalling and interaction and the biochemical languages underlying them are still far from clear despite the huge research input to date.

Arguably one of the critical challenges is the elucidation of the reactions underlying new vascularisation of newly created tissues after implantation or growth induction and the prevention of tissue rejection. Another very interesting and potentially hugely rewarding advance will be the ability to regenerate diseased and damaged nervous tissue. It is now more feasible to envisage a time when spinal damage is reversed through the induced regeneration of, for example, spinal and brain tissue. Currently intractable disease such as Parkinson's and Alzheimer's diseases may be treated by regenerating damaged or missing neural cells. There is a recent report of the successful differentiation *in vitro* of neuronal cells from mouse embryonic stem cells.

Another huge problem is the treatment of immunodeficiency disorders, particularly those that involve the destruction of tissues that produce cells of the immune system. Recently published results seem to hold promise of feasible treatments in the not-too-distant future, e.g. there is a report that infants with severe combined immunodeficiency syndrome (SCID) in the immediate neonatal period have responded to treatment with transplanted stem cells from close blood relatives.

Given the inevitable demands made by research and development technologies, the methods of cell production will need to be scaled up, for example for the mass production of genetically engineered cells. One may envisage a huge clinical demand, e.g. engineered heart, and other muscle cells, pancreatic tissue, skin, bone and other vital organs. New regulatory procedures will evolve out of all this, to ensure quality and reproducibility of manufactured cells, limbs and organs.

There will also be far more collaboration between laboratories through sharing of information, techniques and results. Competition is healthy, but collaboration among research teams will need to increase given the huge, relatively sudden expansion of techniques in this field, coupled with modern financial pressures. It is gratifying to note the active collaboration between the public and private centres that this field of research has opened up, and this collaboration will certainly speed up the development of new biological approaches to disease and organ and tissue replacement.

References

Buckner CD, Epstein RB, Rudolph RH, Clift RA, Storb R, Thomas E D. Allogenic marrow engraftment following whole body irradiation in a patient with leukemia. *Blood* 1970; 35: 741–9.

McCulloch EA, Till JE. The radiation sensitivity of normal mouse bone marrow cells determined by quantitative bone marrow transplantation into irradiated mice. *Radiat Res* 1960; 13: 115–25.

Thomson JA, Itskovitz-Eldor J, Shapiro SS *et al*. Embryonic stem lines derived from human blastocysts. *Science* 1998; 282: 1145–7.

Further reading

Becker AJ, McCulloch EA, Till JE. Cytological demonstration of the clonal nature of spleen colonies derived from transplanted mouse marrow cells. *Nature* 1963; 197: 452–54.

Buerlein MJ, Mckee MD. Calcium sulfates: What's the evidence? *J Orthop Trauma* 2010; 46 (suppl 1): S41.

Evans MJ, Kaufman MH. Establishment in culture of pluripotent cells from mouse embryos. *Nature* 1981; 2982: 154–6.

Kitazawa A, Naka Y, Yamaguchi H, Shimizu N. Accumulation of neurons differentiated from mouse embryonic stem cells in particular areas of culture plate surface. *J Biosci Bioeng* 2010; 110: 238–41.

Lauby AS, Lauby G, Boyer C *et al*. Transplanted BM and BM side population cells contribute progeny to the lung and liver in irradiated mice. *Cytotherapy* 2003; 5: 523–33.

Martin GR. Isolation of a pluripotent cell line from early mouse embryos cultured in medium conditioned by teratocarcinoma stem cells. *Proc Natl Acad Sci USA* 1981; 78: 7634–8.

Mitalipov S, Wolf D. Totipotency, pluripotency and nuclear programming. *Adv Biochem Eng Biotechnol* 2009; 114: 185–99.

Murray JE. Human organ transplantation: background and consequences. *Science* 1992; 256: 1411–16.

Myers LA, Patel DD, Puck JM, Buckley RH. Hematopoietic stem cell transplantation for severe combined immunodeficiency in the neonatal period leads to superior thymic output and improved survival. *Blood* 2002; 99: 872–8.

Schoppy DW, Ruzankina Y, Brown EJ. Removing all obstacles: A critical role for p53 in promoting tissue renewal. *Cell Cycle* 2010; 9. Epub ahead of print.

Till JE, McCulloch EA. Hemopoietic stem cell differentiation. *Biochim Biophys Acta* 1961; 605: 431–59.

Tsigou O, Pomerantseva I, Spencer JA *et al.* Engineered vascularized bone grafts. *Proc Natl Acad Sci USA* 2010; 107: 3311–16.

Ulloa-Montoya F, Verfaillie CM, Hu WS. Culture systems for pluripotent stem cells. *J Biosci Bioeng* 2005; 100: 12–27.

Answers to multiple choice questions

Chapter 1

1	b		4	c
2	d		5	e
3	b		6	c

Chapter 2

1	e		7	b
2	c		8	a
3	d		9	a
4	a		10	d
5	c		11	a
6	a			

Chapter 3

1	d		6	b
2	d		7	a
3	e		8	d
4	b		9	b
5	e			

Chapter 4

1	a		7	c
2	e		8	b
3	d		9	a
4	a		10	e
5	b		11	a
6	b			

Chapter 5

1	c	**4**	b
2	b	**5**	d
3	c	**6**	b

Chapter 6

1	a	**4**	d
2	a	**5**	c
3	c		

Chapter 7

1	b	**4**	b
2	b	**5**	b
3	a		

Glossary

Acquired immunity
immunity acquired from the development of antibodies in response to an antigen, e.g. after having the disease or after vaccination against it

Active immunity
the ability of the body's cells to respond to the antigen, i.e. disease, and produce antibodies directed against the disease antigen

Addison's disease
disease of the adrenal cortex, characterised by skin pigmentation and anaemia due to insufficiency of corticosteroid secretion

Adenocarcinoma
malignant tumour of epithelial tissue; usually originates from glandular tissues

Adenovirus
DNA-based virus responsible for upper respiratory and some eye infections

Adhesion molecule
class of molecules on outer cell membrane surface, mediating cell–cell adhesion and important in the direction of embryonic cell development and differentiation

Adipose tissue
fatty tissue

Adrenocorticotrophin
anterior pituitary hormone that controls the release of, for example, cortisol from the adrenal cortex

Adjuvant
a substance that enhances the activity of another, e.g. the use of chemicals such as aluminium salts to enhance the activity of some vaccines

AIRE
autoimmune regulator; the AIRE gene codes for the thymus autoimmune regulator protein, which is a transcription regulator

Aetiology
study of the causes and characteristics of disease

Allele
alternative forms of genes, only one of which occurs on the same locus of a chromosome

Allergen	substance that can initiate an allergic response, i.e. symptoms of an immune reaction
Allotype	allelic variants of a protein characterised by antigenic differences
ALPS	autoimmune lymphoproliferative syndrome
Anabolic	metabolic changes with, for example, build-up of tissues
Anaphylactic shock	extreme allergic reaction with massive, widespread histamine release resulting in a profound fall in blood pressure and potentially fatal unless promptly treated with adrenaline (epinephrine) to raise blood pressure
ANCA	anti-neutrophil cytoplasmic autoantibody
Anergy	lack of response to an allergen or antigen
Angina pectoris	chest pain during exercise due to inadequacy of coronary oxygen supply
Angiogenesis	formation of blood vessels, stimulated by growth factors and essential for tumorigenesis and tumour growth; therefore a target for development of anti-cancer drugs
Angiostasis	physiological regulation of new blood vessel biosynthesis – a strictly controlled system
Ankylosing spondylitis	inflammation of the synovial joints in the spinal column
Anterolateral	in front of the body and away from the midline
Anthrax	acute infectious disease of farm animals caused by *Bacillus anthracis*; can be transmitted to humans, causing potentially fatal lesions in lungs and skin
Antibody	lymphocyte-produced protein directed against and which neutralises a specific antigen
Antigen	substance, usually large, e.g. a protein, identified by the organism as foreign, and which evokes an immune response
Atherosclerosis	arterial disease with deposition of fatty plaques on the endothelial wall, resulting in potentially dangerous narrowing of the lumen
Attenuated vaccine	live pathogens that have lost their virulence but are still capable of inducing a protective immune response to the virulent forms of the pathogen, e.g. Sabin polio vaccine. Methods and reagents used include alum precipitation, formaldehyde and heating

Autoantibody	antibody created against a component, e.g. a protein of the same organism
Autoimmunity	disease produced when the autoimmune system fails to recognise part of itself and attacks that tissue or organ
Bacteriophage	a virus able to penetrate and reproduce multiple copies of itself within another cell, e.g. a bacterium
Basement membrane	thin layer of connective tissue supporting, usually, a layer or layers of epithelium
Biological drug	medicinal preparation based on a naturally occurring biological chemical structure (USA: biologic drug or biologic)
Biosynthesis	synthesis of anything by a living organism
BNF	*British National Formulary*
Blue tongue disease	a viral disease of sheep and cattle, characterised by fever and catarrh
BSE	bovine spongiform encephalopathy; a neurodegenerative and fatal disease of the brain, which becomes spongy with plaque formation
Carcinogenesis	transformation of healthy cells, tissues or organs into cancerous cells, tissues or organs
CD cell	cluster of differentiation cell
Chemokine	peptide or protein that is released by inflamed cells; mediates inflammation by attracting white blood cells to an inflamed areas
Chemotaxis	migration or movement, usually of cells, which are attracted to a particular chemical stimulus
Chimaeric	here, a molecule or structure composed of two or more parts of different origin
Cloning	here, creation of an identical genetic copy of a parent, i.e. the same genome, e.g. Dolly the Sheep
Codon	functional triplet of deoxynucleotides in the genome coding, ultimately for an amino acid; some codons provide functional signals, e.g. the STOP codon
Colitis	inflammation of the colon
Congenital	referring to an inherited characteristic or condition

Contagion	transmission of disease through direct contact with an infected person (or other animal)
CRH	corticotrophin-releasing hormone
Cytokine	protein or peptide released by the cell in response to antigenic activation of the cell
Cytotoxic	toxic to cellular tissue
Double helix	with respect to DNA, a spiral formed by the cross-linking of the DNA bases adenine–thymine (A–T) and cytosine–guanine (C–G)
DR	death receptor
Endogenous	naturally occurring within the organism
Endothelium	single layer of inner lining cells of the cardiovascular system
Extrachromosomal	occurring or existing outside the chromosomal influence or input
Exudative	flowing or oozing of fluids from the tissues
FoxP3	(forkhead box protein 3), named after a gene originally described in *Drosophila* sp., encodes a transcription–repressor protein in the immune system
Gag protein	protein of nucleoplasmid shell that surrounds the retroviral RNA
Gene	DNA sequence that codes for, for example, a protein or for a characteristic of the phenotype
Gene knock-out	functional elimination or inactivation of a specific gene, by either physical removal or alteration of the gene
Genetic code	the biological rules whereby a DNA sequence codes, ultimately, for a specific protein or for an instruction governing the activity of the enzyme RNA polymerase
Genetic engineering	the science of recombinant DNA technology
Genome	the genetic database of an individual of the species, made up of the orderly sequence of genes
Genotype	genetic constitution of, for example, a cell, an organ or the individual member of a defined species
GIT	gastrointestinal tract
Glomerulonephritis	disease of the kidney glomeruli that impairs filtration, through, for example, antigen–antibody complex precipitates

Gluconeogenesis	biosynthesis of glucose from non-carbohydrate precursors
Glycosylation	chemical reaction linking glycosides (e.g. sugars) to other moieties, e.g. proteins
G-protein	member of the guanine nucleotide-binding proteins that mediate post-receptor cascades in the cell membrane
Granulocytes	group of white blood cells that stain with the Romanovsky stain; according to the colour of stain are classified as basophils, eosinophils or neutrophils
GWAS	genome-wide association studies
Haematopoietic	pertaining to the creation of blood
Haemolytic	causing destruction of red blood cells
Hapten	a relatively small molecule that is able, when linked to a larger molecule, e.g. a protein, to provoke an immune response
Herpes simplex virus	infective agent for, for example, cold sores
HIV	human immunodeficiency virus
Humoral	adjective describing anything e.g. cells circulating in the bloodstream
Hyperthermia	raised body temperature
Hypothermia	lowered body temperature
IFN-α	interferon-α
Integrase	retrovirus enzyme that catalyses the integration of the viral genome into that of the host
Interferons	group of glycoproteins produced by cells infected with viruses; they block viral replication in the infected cell
Interleukins	class of proteins secreted principally by T lymphocytes and macrophages, and that induce differentiation and growth of haematopoietic stem cells and lymphocytes
IRF	interferon regulatory factor
Knockout mice	a mouse that has been genetically engineered so that one or more of its genes has been deleted or switched off using genetic engineering techniques
K-*ras*	an oncogene, the mutations of which are critically important in carcinogenesis, notably in colorectal, lung and pancreatic cancers

Leukocyte	white blood cell with amoeboid properties, i.e. ability to ingest and inactivate particles, e.g. bacteria
Ligand	any molecule that binds, usually non-covalently, to another molecule, e.g. TNF-α, is the ligand that binds to its receptor on the cell membrane
Liposome	microscopic sphere composed of an aqueous inner core surrounded by a lipophilic outer shell; a pharmaceutical delivery system for, for example, drugs
Lymphoid trafficking	movement of lymphocytes in response to mediators of inflammation
Lymphokine	chemical mediator of inflammation produced by lymphocytes
Macrophage	phagocytic white cell scavenger that ingests foreign cells and bacteria
Macule	highly circumscribed, flat patch of skin depigmentation (see also Vitiligo)
Malignancy	with regard to medicine, a cancer with potential for or actual invasion of healthy tissues
Mast cell	large cell situated in connective tissue that releases inflammatory mediators, e.g. histamine and 5-hydroxytryptamine (5-HT)
Metastasis	spread of a tumour from its site of formation to distant tissues
Morphoea	form of localised scleroderma, usually confined to skin, with slow resolution of symptoms
Multiple sclerosis	chronic autoimmune nervous system disorder caused by progressive demyelination of nerves; thymus failure may be causative
Murine	adjective with reference to mice
Mutation	change in the genetic make-up of an organism; may be caused by, for example, irradiation or chemical action
Myasthenia gravis	autoimmune disease with muscle paralysis due to destruction of the neuromuscular junction
Negative feedback	describing a self-regulatory system whereby the end-point, e.g. product of a biochemical chemical reaction, can switch off further production of itself by the enzymes involved
Neoplasm	abnormal new growth; in a clinical context usually refers to a tumour

Noxious	harmful; injurious to the health of the organism
Nucleoplasmid	part of a retrovirus that contains its RNA genome and the integrase enzyme
Oligodendrocyte	a central nervous cell that insulates axons
Paramyxovirus	airborne virus transmitting, for example, measles
Pasteurisation	use of heat to achieve incomplete or partial sterilisation of any substance in order to inactivate microorganisms within that substance
PCR	polymerase chain reaction
Phenotype	characteristics of one individual within a genotype
Polymorphism	in genetics, occurrence of more than one form of a chromosome, with consequent occurrence of more than one morphological type within a given population of that species
Positive feedback	describing a self-regulatory system whereby the end-point, e.g. the release of luteinising hormone from the anterior pituitary gland, is greatly increased through the hormone estradiol just before ovulation
Polynucleotide	a nucleotide chain consisting of 13 or more nucleotides
Posthumous	after death
PR3	proteinase 3, an enzyme involved in vasculitis
Prenatal	before birth
Proteomics	discipline devoted to the study of the complete set of proteins produced by a given genome
Psoriasis	chronic, autoimmune disease of the skin with formation of pink, scaly patch-like lesions on the skin and scalp
Purine	an organic base; adenine and guanine are purines
Pyrimidine	an organic base; cytosine and thymine are pyrimidines
RA	rheumatoid arthritis
rAAV virus	non-pathogenic virus of *Parvoviridae* virus family; of interest as therapeutic vectors
Recombinant	in DNA technology, an engineered DNA sequence
Restriction enzymes (restriction endonucleases)	enzymes that cut single or double-stranded DNA only at points specific for the enzyme

Retrovirus a virus containing RNA and the enzyme reverse transcriptase; this virus can penetrate a cell and convert its RNA to DNA, which is then incorporated into the host DNA

Reverse transcriptase enzyme that catalyses the conversion of RNA into the corresponding DNA; found in retroviruses

Rheumatoid factor an autoantibody raised against the patient's IgG by the immune system; the autoantibody can provoke an inflammatory reaction; patients with rheumatoid arthritis may test positive for rheumatoid factor

Ribosome a cytoplasmic protein composed of subunits that bind to mRNA and translate its nucleotide sequence into the corresponding amino acids, which it then forms into the protein

Serendipity with respect to science, a phenomenon of research that is a fortunate and sometimes unplanned discovery

SLE systemic lupus erythematosus

SNP single nucleotide polymorphism

Splice to cut a nucleotide or protein chain at a defined point, often for the experimental purpose of adding to, substituting or deleting, for example, amino acids or nucleotides from a chain of these

Stochastic governed by chance

Synovial relating to the synovial fluid in the joint

T cell T lymphocyte

TCR T-cell receptor

T-helper cell (Th) T cell that helps other cells of the immune system recognise and to respond to antigens; they secrete cytokines which activate B and T cells, thereby boosting antibody production

Thymectomy removal of the thymus gland

TNF-α tumour necrosis factor-α

Transcription transfer of genetic information from DNA to RNA

Trauma in physiological terms, injury or shock to a tissue or system

Vaccine an antigenic preparation derived from a disease-carrying organism that will stimulate the recipient body to develop specific antibodies to it and thereby confer active immunity against the disease

Vasculitis	inflammation of blood vessels through autoimmune attack by white blood cells
Vector	in molecular biology, a carrier of an amino acid or nucleotide sequence, e.g. a plasmid or virus
Vitiligo	autoimmune disease causing skin depigmentation; characterised by occurrence of white macules or patches on the skin; more prevalent in dark-skinned individuals
Wnt signalling pathway	a pathway involved in many different biochemical reactions, e.g. in embryogenesis, driven by the *Wnt* gene

Reference

Concise Colour Oxford Dictionary, 2nd edn. oxford: Oxford University Press.

Index